JAN DE VRIES was born in 1937 in Holland and grew up during the difficult war years in occupied territory. Although he graduated in pharmacy, he soon turned to alternative medicine. His most influential teacher was Dr Alfred Vogel in Switzerland, and they have worked together closely for 35 years.

In 1970 he and his family moved to Scotland and settled on the west coast in Troon, where he set up a residential clinic called Mokoia. He also has clinics in Newcastle, Edinburgh and London. Since 1990 he has been involved in Klein Vink in Arcen, Holland, doing research into the efficacy of herbal medicine for the European Commission.

He lectures throughout the world and is a regular broadcaster on BBC radio.

MULTIPLE SCLEROSIS

Books available by the same author

By Appointment Only series:

Stress and Nervous Disorders (3rd impression)
Traditional Home and Herbal Remedies (5th impression)
Arthritis, Rheumatism and Psoriasis (5th impression)
The Miracle of Life (2nd impression)
Neck and Back Problems (4th impression)
Migraine and Epilepsy (3rd impression)
Cancer and Leukemia (2nd impression)
Viruses, Allergies and the Immune System (4th impression)
Realistic Weight Control (2nd impression)
Who's Next?
Heart and Blood Circulatory Problems
Asthma and Bronchitis
Life Without Arthritis — The Maori Way
Skin Diseases

Nature's Gift series:

Body Energy (2nd impression)
Water — Healer or Poison?
Food

Well Woman series:
Menstrual and Pre-menstrual Tension

MULTIPLE SCLEROSIS

JAN DE VRIES

MAINSTREAM
PUBLISHING

This edition 1992
First published in Great Britain 1985, reprinted 1987 and 1989, by
MAINSTREAM PUBLISHING COMPANY (EDINBURGH) LTD
7 Albany Street
Edinburgh EH1 3UG

ISBN 0 906391 98 9 (paper)

A catalogue record for this book is available from the British Library

Reproduced from disc in 11/12pt Andover by Mainstream Publishing
Printed in Great Britain by Billings & Sons Ltd, Worcester

Contents

Foreword

I FIND it uniquely pleasant to be connected with a book on methods of controlling Multiple Sclerosis. Thirty-five years ago I was solemnly informed, by no less a person than the President of the Multiple Sclerosis Society himself, that I should prepare for the end. My condition, in his opinion, was beyond hope. And a pitiable condition indeed it most certainly was. No-one looking at me — unable to walk, to balance myself, to stand up, to see to any purpose, to talk clearly, to pick up a pen even, far less to write — would have questioned his opinion. But I am stubborn. And though others may have agreed with him (and who's to blame them?) I disagreed violently. I had my helpless carcass removed from the Queen Square Hospital by my loving wife and brought home. What happened then, I explain later in a lecture I gave in The Netherlands (see chapter 2). But before I leave you to read the book in peace, I have a few observations to make about its author.

Jan de Vries and I first met when he arranged that I should give a lecture in Amsterdam — with Jan himself translating it into Dutch — a language of which I am totally ignorant.

7

Then began an association which has lasted now for 12 years. It is based, I think, on a mutual respect. I respect him, for the breadth of his knowledge and his constant endeavour to widen it by studying different techniques in many different countries. He respects me, for reacting positively to the expert prediction of my imminent death, taking my future into my own hands, analysing my problem correctly and then solving it.

Our opinions meet in the realisation that there is no one and only way to control Multiple Sclerosis (or any other degenerative "disease"), no one and only cause, no one and only way to help even one individual. Certain guidelines appear to be applicable to most people who are degeneratives. (Since we are all degenerating, after a certain age — that being the price for living — I should perhaps refer to people who are degenerating too quickly.) I soon became aware that the regimen which had helped me, also helped a great variety of other people in that unfortunate category.

The fact that the correct diet helped not only Multiple Sclerosis sufferers, but also victims of other degenerative complaints, was first brought to my attention quite fortuitously.

A lady, who had put her husband on my regimen, rang up to say she wanted to come to London to visit me. As she intended to drive well over 100 miles, I tried to dissuade her, but she wouldn't listen. When she arrived the following day, it was to present me with a bottle of brandy and a huge basket of flowers, like the ones that stand beside filmstars on gala occasions. I was completely taken aback. "Don't tell me your husband has begun to improve already," I said. "It's not my husband," she replied. "It's me. My arthritis has gone completely."

This is the story that emerged. Her husband had said the regime would be too horrible to follow. To encourage him to persevere, she joined him in following the diet strictly. And in the event her arthritis had vanished (physical problems clear up more quickly than do nerve problems).

What does this have to do with Jan de Vries? Not much, I suppose, except that it illustrates the sort of gratitude we both evoke from those we help. I can't speak for Jan, of course, but personally, over a period of fifteen years or so, I have helped clear up almost every degenerative "disease" in the book.

The case that is perhaps most outstanding is that of a composer, whom I first met in Santa Monica, Los Angeles. He was in hospital and on a breathing machine twenty-four hours a day. His problem was Amyotrophic Lateral Sclerosis, known there as Lou Gering's disease, after a famous baseball player who died of it and known in Britain also as Motor Neurone Disease.

I had been taken to see him by his sister, a screen-writing friend, who told me that he was in danger of being taken off his life support machine. Five doctors had met that morning, she told me, to decide on his future, and the vote had gone three to two against him. Quite understandably — there are queues of deserving cases waiting to be helped and he had had his time. His own doctor had argued so persuasively on his behalf that he had been granted a "stay of execution".

At that point I took over. He had money and was in a private room with a male nurse and also had his own fridge. I threw out the junk that was in there and stocked it with the appropriate foods. Then I had a long talk with his nurse.

A few months later, he was back home and on his machine only at nights. He acquired a secretary with a knowledge of music to whom he could dictate and began work again. Before I left America (three years ago) he had already published two records of groups of songs. I had a letter a week or so ago, telling me that he is still busily at work. Significantly too, since I last saw him he was hospitalised with pneumonia and came through unscathed.

Anyone who knows the customary course of this "disease" — down and out in a year or so — will have to admit that something remarkable was achieved.

I report this case in detail, though I'm writing a foreword to a book by Jan de Vries. I know he has had many similar experiences, but they cannot carry conviction at second hand. This is the sort of triumph that Jan has accomplished and he has done it time and time again. It is for Jan himself to tell you of them and to explain, in wiser language than mine, the various methods he has adopted.

Roger MacDougall

Preface

A FEW years ago I attended a lecture where a medical doctor spoke on the subject of Multiple Sclerosis. He stated that he could give thirteen possible reasons for Multiple Sclerosis but that we have to compare this disease to an Agatha Christie thriller and find the answer to the mystery on the last page. However, he went on to say that the answer had not been found yet.

Listening attentively to him while he listed the thirteen possible causes, I never heard him mention the word "diet", which created the impression that Multiple Sclerosis as a degenerative disease and diet were not interconnected.

During question time I asked him whether he thought that there was no connection between Multiple Sclerosis and diet. He replied that there was absolutely no relation, but that he had heard of people who stressed the importance of a dietary connection. These people, however, were only interested in making money out of this particular affliction. I could not help but inform him that when I studied acupuncture in China, I did not come across Multiple Sclerosis cases. Unfortunately, to my great surprise, visiting Taiwan a couple of years ago to attend a congress in the city of Taipei, I was slightly surprised to be asked to give a lecture on this subject.

I asked the organisers on my arrival for the reason behind their choice of subject and was told that Multiple Sclerosis used not to be a problem there, but unfortunately nowadays it was. One of the Chinese professors blamed the convenience foods as well as the foods imported from the West into Taiwan.

In a way I was quite happy to hear this, as I had always felt that diet had so much bearing on this dreadful disease. When I told the lecturer about this particular incident he responded by saying that China was a great distance away. I suggested we stay nearer home and look at the geographical distribution of Multiple Sclerosis and relate this to the intake of foods rich in linoleic acid or fatty acids, such as fish.

If we look at the Faroe Islands, we see that there is a very low incidence of Multiple Sclerosis. The Faroe Islanders have a Danish genetic background and remained fishermen. In our own Shetland Islands, however, a drastic change in diet took place, in line with the agricultural influence from Britain. With the British diet, the Shetland Islanders acquired the British incidence of Multiple Sclerosis. Similarities are noticeable in the Netherlands and in Scandinavian countries.

Although Multiple Sclerosis occurs in most western countries, with a higher incidence in the cities, we cannot underestimate the fact that the highest percentage of Multiple Sclerosis is noted in the Orkneys and Shetlands in northern Scotland. In these particular areas, occurrence of Multiple Sclerosis is three times higher than in the rest of the UK, followed by New York City, which has the second highest rate in the world. It is also interesting to see that the intake of fat in the north of Scotland is 19% greater than elsewhere in the United Kingdom and, of course, one cannot forget the fact that the intake of alcoholic drinks is very high in Scotland.

It is a fact that incidence of Multiple Sclerosis is low in tropical countries. This would appear not to relate so much to the temperature as to dietary management.

In 1960 a lady consulted us in our clinic in The Netherlands. She had made a remarkable recovery, on a diet designed by Dr Evers from Germany. When I examined the diet regime I noticed that the advised fat-intake was very low. Large amounts of fresh fruit, fresh vegetables and grains were recommended. From that time on we treated Multiple Sclerosis according to the Dr Evers methods and we achieved a certain measure of success.

After having settled in Britain about fifteen years ago, a lady-patient informed me that she had been following the Roger MacDougall diet. She followed his instructions carefully and had improved quite considerably. Of course I was interested in her story and wrote to Roger MacDougall. He immediately replied with the message that he felt like a caller in the wilderness. After a lot of research and then strictly adhering to a gluten free diet, he had achieved great success in his own management of the disease. Any assistance in establishing his diet and views would be most welcome.

I went to see him shortly after, on a visit to London, and could not believe my ears when I heard him running down the stairs. When he opened the front door, I found myself looking at a most active person and the thought immediately arose that if this man had spent a period of more than twenty years in a wheelchair, a miracle must have happened. After a long conversation with him I came to the conclusion that this man did not just have a remission; the credit for his present condition must largely be ascribed to his dietary regime.

Later on I had to go and see some Dutch patients who stayed in the Hilton Hotel and as we found we still had so much to discuss, he decided to come along with me. Both of us walked the length of Piccadilly and his step was faster than mine.

My curiosity about his methods was aroused and I decided to do some double tests. I put a group of people on the Evers diet and another group on the MacDougall diet. Undoubtedly the last group made more progress than the first group and since that time, working along the lines of this dietary regime, some surprising successes have been achieved.

I do hope that from the following chapters Multiple Sclerosis sufferers will gain a little more enlightenment and will also learn the importance of eating the proper food. Several other methods which will help their condition are also described.

However, let there be no misunderstanding: Multiple Sclerosis is NOT curable. Let me quote Roger MacDougall on that point: "As well try to cure a Chinaman of being Chinese. I was born a Sclerotic. It's in my genes. It's the hand I was dealt at conception with which to play out the game of life. Short of genetic engineering, I will die a Sclerotic. But I have lived a symptom-free life for more than fifteen years, except for a few brief lapses when I have been foolish enough and indulgent enough to break the rules. If I mistreat my body, it responds by renewing the old familiar symptoms — weirdly in exactly the reverse order in which they vanished. First to return is a touch of nystagmus (the last to go), then comes a slight paralysis in my right hand — my worst hand when I was crippled and the second last symptom to clear up. I've never dared to go on misbehaving and find out what would happen next."

The important point then is that Multiple Sclerosis,

though not curable by present drug dependent medical methods, IS CONTROLLABLE.

1

What is Multiple Sclerosis?

A FEW years ago I was asked to give a lecture on Multiple Sclerosis for an international congress. The possible causes of it, what really was Multiple Sclerosis and in what way could it be diagnosed. I informed my listeners that while treating the problem over the last twenty-five years, I had found several times that Multiple Sclerosis had been wrongly diagnosed. We should, therefore, be careful not to label a patient with Multiple Sclerosis as soon as certain possible symptoms occur. Proper testing and investigations should always be carried out. I also said that it was easy to place a patient with symptoms which are difficult to diagnose under the umbrella of Multiple Sclerosis.

Immediately after I had finished this lecture, the well known neurologist, Dr Sanchez Perez from Spain, stood up. To my great surprise he fully agreed with this statement and said that this mistake was made too often. This brings us to the questions: what really is Multiple Sclerosis and is there an answer to the problem?

As we know, Multiple Sclerosis is a disease of the

nervous system where the protective sheath of the nerve fibre suffers damage. This, of course, can result in some very nasty physical symptoms.

First we see that muscle co-ordination is affected throughout the whole body, speech impediment can occur, loss of balance, co-ordination movements of hands and limbs and double vision. Often these problems become progressively worse.

Very often Multiple Sclerosis will start with small sensations — it can be a little dizziness or perhaps some pins and needles, as it is often described, or tiredness and fatigue.

The name Multiple Sclerosis means "many scars". It is a slowly progressive disease that is characterised by disseminated patches of demyelination in the central nervous system. This results in multiple and varied neurologic symptoms and signs, usually with periods of remission and exacerbations. Women are affected somewhat more often than men.

The disease is very difficult to diagnose accurately, as it mimics many other neuro-muscular disorders. The symptoms are related to the site of demyelination. The periods of remission occur when the signs and symptoms are less troublesome or may even disappear completely. These periods of remission can last for weeks, months or even years.

In laymen's terms it is often said that we should see Multiple Sclerosis as a localised insulation breakdown. When the myelin sheath on certain parts suffers damage, problems usually occur. With Multiple Sclerosis patients we find that damage to the nerve sheath may possibly be caused by severe trauma. There are a few schools of thought about this reasoning, including differences of opinion as to the cause of the trauma that triggered it off in the first instance.

Some say that the disease is a result of an auto-immune response. Others say that it can be a problem of the metabolic system, while still others take it for granted that the disease comes from a virus or an infection. Let us be honest, if we put one thousand Multiple Sclerosis patients in a line, we will find that every one of these thousand patients is different and whatever the cause might be, one has to treat each patient individually. One cannot put a Multiple Sclerosis patient on a set programme until the background of this patient is known.

When interviewing Multiple Sclerosis patients one receives the most varying answers to the usual questions. When asked what the first symptoms were, some will answer double vision, some say that it felt like walking on a floor of jelly and some describe it as like walking on snow, where other patients started off with bladder problems.

Going into the background of Multiple Sclerosis patients and treating the patient as an individual, we come to several possible reasons why the patient became a victim of Multiple Sclerosis.

With a possible viral infection there is no doubt that consequent lymphocyte sensitivity has attacked the auto-immune process. When patients suffering from measles are being treated with homoeopathic remedies we very often hear complaints about similar symptoms. Small dental or throat infections could possibly be the trigger that starts the disease. For that reason it is very important to find out everything about the background of the patient: when and where the first symptoms started, what kind of symptoms the patient first suffered and how it all happened. The necessity of good investigation in search of the cause of Multiple Sclerosis is therefore very important and in treating that cause some surprising results have been achieved.

Observations that Multiple Sclerosis might be related to

the amount of fat in the diet and to the deficiency of poly-unsaturated fatty acids, have been proven in many cases to be quite true, especially in Scotland. It is claimed that the incidence of Multiple Sclerosis in Scotland is three times higher than elsewhere in the world. Treating patients in Scotland on a special dietary regime has given hope to many patients.

Linoleic acid, which is a very important poly-unsaturated fat, very often given in the form of sunflowerseed-oil, safflowerseed-oil or Oil of Evening Primrose, has shown that the lymphocyte attack on the brain has slowed down the deterioration of this particular process. It is often said that there is a low incidence of Multiple Sclerosis in tropical countries because these oils are taken as part of the daily diet.

Another possible reason for Multiple Sclerosis, mostly occurring between the age of twenty to forty-five is that stress or too rich living could accelerate the degenerative process of this metabolic disease.

I am always filled with great sympathy when seeing patients who have been diagnosed as suffering from Multiple Sclerosis. Sometimes they have been told that they have a problem which they have to learn to live with and to accept that there is no reason, or cure. These patients often go home in despair and look up their medical dictionaries to find that most tell them that the cause is unknown. They will read that the insulation of the nerves has deteriorated, that paralysis, partial blindness, lack of balance will occur. They gain a lot of knowledge regarding this problem, but very little hope. These particular patients will become more and more stressed and stress is a great enemy to the Multiple Sclerosis patient. These people should be approached in a positive way and given help where possible.

Let us be very honest about one thing, and that is that

Multiple Sclerosis CANNOT BE CURED. What is dead remains dead, but there is hope from past research and experiences from Multiple Sclerosis patients who have found that it is a controllable disease and that although the destroyed myelin sheaths of the fibres will never recover, by taking a positive dietary and supplement approach, some really surprising results have been obtained.

Even if one part of the brain might be damaged the function of that part might be taken over by other parts. This is often seen as a remission. Some of these bypass routes should be further researched and developed with Multiple Sclerosis patients. It is advisable to inform Multiple Sclerosis patients in all honesty what their problem entails and that a positive approach is vital. Several methods which have been a blessing to many, are discussed in this book.

There is no doubt that the orthodox drug treatment used in degenerative diseases gives relief. Unfortunately this is only temporary. Another method used is manipulation, although I would suggest that a much better method is the preventative approach.

A good dietary regime is of paramount importance. As a Multiple Sclerosis sufferer himself, Professor Roger MacDougall came to this conclusion many years ago. He thought perhaps a possible infection or a mysterious virus was the cause and considered that there might be a chemical imbalance in his system. Bringing this train of thought to its logical conclusion he therefore designed a diet, used by people in those days when there was no known Multiple Sclerosis.

He started out from the fact that in my own country, The Netherlands, during the war no coeliac diseases occurred, as, out of necessity, the intake of gluten products was nearly zero. He also thought that in a sugar-free diet there is an indication that diabetes or hypoglycaemia is very low or non-existent, as is the case with a diet free of milkfats in relation to cardio-vascular problems. Following this way of thinking he came to the right conclusion, which is backed up by his present state of health.

For all the patients who have asked what Multiple Sclerosis is or what the cause of it is, I feel that Roger MacDougall's answer to Multiple Sclerosis, researched by himself as well as by many other researchers and scientists, has been of great help.

With pleasure and satisfaction I look back on a lecture we gave together in The Netherlands in 1975. I think of all the people who, after that particular lecture, have been using the Roger MacDougall system. Some have had great success.

I would like to repeat that particular lecture in the next chapter, as I am of the opinion that it fully explains Roger MacDougall's approach to the problem. He logically and sensibly set about solving the difficulties created by this disease and gave many patients who had lost hope for the future a new lease of life.

From years of experience treating these patients, I have come to the honest conclusion that although Multiple Sclerosis is not curable, it is controllable, and even though I do not like to give anybody false hopes, at the same time I would like to stress the importance of positive thought, as I have found this to be most beneficial.

2

The Netherlands Lecture

WHAT FOLLOWS in this chapter is largely the text of the joint lecture given by myself and Roger MacDougall, a Multiple Sclerosis sufferer.

Twenty years ago I was in a fairly terminal condition of Multiple Sclerosis. Now I am totally symptom-free. That in itself does not justify my presence. All of you have no doubt known of remissions — some even perhaps as remarkable as mine.

Why I feel I'm entitled to be here is because the regimen which in my opinion caused my remission appears to have the same happy effect on so many others who try it and stick to it faithfully over a sufficiently long period of time.

Recently I sent out a circular asking routine questions of a small number of people who had tried my method, and written to say that they found it helped. I wanted to know if the improvement was being maintained, and a gratifyingly large majority of the replies came from people continuing to improve and determined to stick rigidly to what they believe to be their way back to health.

Am I suggesting then that when I decided to leave my neurologists eighteen years ago, and seek my own way back to health, I found some answer which my neurologists should have found for me? Not really.

What I am suggesting is that to call Multiple Sclerosis a neurological disease is exactly like calling Scarlet Fever a skin disease, and that expecting a neurologist to understand and treat it, is like expecting a dermatologist to cope with Scarlet Fever.

I think it is because it is thought to be a problem for neurologists to solve that Multiple Sclerosis has baffled all attempts to deal with it. It is not in my mind a problem with which a neurologist's training in any way qualifies him to cope. It is a problem, not of disease, but of inadequate cell tissue renewal.

I think I have attained a state of 100% symptom-free health by finding out how to restore to my metabolism its natural recuperative power, its ability to build healthy cell tissue once more for its myelin sheath.*

Your immediate reaction to my claim may be to say I am experiencing a remission. My response is to agree. Of course I am experiencing a remission. I am totally symptom-free but I am not cured. I am still a sclerotic just as a diabetic is still a diabetic even when his symptoms are totally

---

* It is many years since I wrote this lecture. Rereading it, I find only one point on which I would like to enlarge.

I attribute my recovery to the restoration of the myelin sheath of my nervous system. While this may be so, I realise that there is an alternative explanation. Apparently we have a massive superfluity of neurons and it is possible that some of these may have taken over from the damaged ones.

Roger MacDougall

controlled.

You, of course, may go further and say I am experiencing an inexplicable remission. Now I disagree. To me there is obviously no such thing as an inexplicable remission. There must be an explanation for any event in a causally connected universe. What is meant is that it is a remission which medicine cannot explain. And with this, of course, I have to agree.

I think, you see, that I was lucky enough to find the true explanation precisely because I am not a doctor and followed a path which the rules and practices of medicine could not conceivably have allowed me to embark on.

I am certain that I am experiencing a self-induced remission and I am also certain that I found out how to achieve this, not because I studied medicine, but paradoxically, because I did *not* study medicine, because I looked at my problem completely from scratch, without making any assumptions, without taking anything for granted, without any preconceived ideas. The only assumption I made was that medicine had failed to find an answer, so I had better try elsewhere.

Where else to try? Obviously, at the beginning. And what is the beginning? The beginning has to be life itself.

So I began reading Heinz Woltereck's *The Miracle of Life*. I began, in other words, by studying not medicine, but biochemistry. And what is Life? Life is a biochemical process — the process of constant cell renewal. A living being is endless, continuous bio-chemical activity. The raw materials of this activity are the chemicals ingested as food and drink. What is needed to sustain the process of healthy cell renewal is abstracted from the raw material and the rest is excreted.

Here, I thought, we will perhaps find the answer to the cause of all degenerative "diseases". In every so-called degenerative disease, a constant characteristic would appear to be the inability of the metabolism to carry on creating an adequate supply of healthy replacement cell tissue.

Why doesn't the body create this essential substance? Does it have to be because it is being attacked by some disease mechanism? Could it not be that it is simply not being supplied with the necessary raw materials?

If it is possible for you to do it, I would like you all at this point to forget that you are doctors. Forget all the preconceived ideas which you take for granted and think of yourselves as intelligent laymen. Forget everything you have been taught and everything you have been told and accept only what you know and can demonstrate pragmatically, from actual experience and not from hearsay.

The first thing which struck me anew when I read Heinz Woltereck's *The Miracle of Life* was something I'd known and accepted and never really thought about — this fact that life is the constant renewal of cell tissue. It is something we all know. That is what we all are — not sort of living cadavers, but chemical processes.

And what was "degenerative disease" (as I've said I was assuming that Multiple Sclerosis came into that category)? "Degenerative disease" was the exact opposite. The slow breakdown or degeneration of cell tissue.

Perhaps it was wrong, I felt, to look on Multiple Sclerosis as a disease in which something was attacking the body. Perhaps it was wrong to think that something — be it germ, virus or bacillus or whatever — had in its turn to be attacked.

Perhaps Multiple Sclerosis should be regarded simply as a breakdown in the chemical process of life. Perhaps what was needed was not that the body should be subjected to powerful drugs, but that it should be helped and encouraged to build new replacement tissue — as simple as that.

If life is the renewal of our cell tissue, so degenerative "disease" is our failure to renew it. In *Act of Creation* Arthur Koestler refers to the juxtaposition of two matrices not previously connected, but suddenly seen to be related as the original concept of a discovery. Funnily enough he describes the exact situation in which I find myself as an innovator, fighting the inertia of a dogmatically entrenched Establishment. But before I can expect the establishment to come round to my way of thinking I have to come up with something more tangible than a theory. It may be true that the victim of Multiple Sclerosis, for instance, simply has to be enabled to build new cell tissue. But how to do this?

The first hint came to me from a discovery made in The Netherlands. Two Dutch physicians were the first to realise that the way to remove the symptoms of coeliac disease was to remove the gluten from the diet. With gluten removed, the individual resumes the process of building healthy tissue for the damaged mucosal lining of the upper bowel. (Incidentally, it is significant to notice that a coeliac is not cured any more than I am or a diabetic is, but simply controlled.)

What else? I looked around for other similar degenerative conditions which are perhaps not in any real sense diseases and which are improved or removed by cutting out some element in the diet. The most obvious were diabetes and hypoglycaemia which are improved by the removal of sugar from the diet.

The other obvious candidate for removal was dairy cream whose absence seems to help those with cardio-vascular conditions. I cut out cereals, sugar and milk fat and now began to think more logically about the problem of nutrition. Obviously, in removing these three foodstuffs I was removing much more from my diet than the offending ingredients. By removing cereals I was not only removing gluten but also my principal source of the B-group of vitamins.

I realised that to remain healthy I would have to make good this loss. Similarly by removing milk-fat, I was losing, among other things, calcium. In this rather haphazard way I built up the concept that in order to follow the diet I felt to be necessary, I had to enrich it with a supplement of vitamins and minerals.

Five years ago when I could run upstairs two at a time, I thought I had reached the peak of my recovery. But it is only two years since I found I could run downstairs two at a time again. Incredible though it may seem, I am still improving.

All this time I was accepting advice from a variety of sympathetic doctors and nutritionists. Also I was helped by a biochemist in Aberdeen who had written to the *Lancet* of his improvement while on my therapy and helped me improve the supplement still further.

I had now begun to read again and in these ways I arrived at the vitamin/mineral supplement which I now advocate.

By following the diet I had now defined and adding to it this vitamin/mineral supplement, many hundreds of people appear to be controlling the symptoms of their Multiple Sclerosis and getting better slowly.

Why should this be so? Neurologists look for the reason behind my success by conducting medical tests and all the time they find nothing. To my way of thinking this is because the tests they apply are quite inapplicable. They use the so-called double-blind trial with placebo.

It seems obvious to me at least that this method cannot produce meaningful results unless there is only one variable. With diet this is impossible.

This type of test is useful only for testing a *drug*. One group gets the drug — the other gets the placebo. The results can then be reasonably compared.

With a diet things are quite different. For one thing it is impossible to test only one ingredient. Take the polyunsaturated fats for example. Their effectiveness varies with the amount of anti-oxidant present in the patient. Without it the polyunsaturated fats are broken down prematurely. And I don't see how the amount of anti-oxidant in an individual can be accurately measured. It doesn't just depend on what dosage of Vitamin E or Vitamin C he has received for instance. It depends on how much other food he has eaten and how rich that was in Vitamin E and C, and also on the efficiency of his particular metabolism.

I'd hate to be a researcher trying to work that one out, trying to find out what percentage of the long-chain carbon molecules in the polyunsaturated fats finally got through in their pristine long-chain form. Similarly it is believed that the presence of magnesium is necessary if B1 is to be metabolised.

And how can you test the effect of Vitamin B12 by giving one group B12, by injection or orally, and giving another group a placebo? Someone in the second group may have a liver-pâté sandwich as a snack or grilled liver for lunch and ingest more B12 than anyone in the first group. Similarly with other vitamins and minerals. You'd even have to analyse and measure the chemical content of the water or beer or whatever liquid anyone drank.

A test of this sort is quite an impractical project, and it has certainly never been done, though I've seen it stated time and again by neurologists who should know better that my method has been tested. As I've just shown there is no conceivable way in which this can be true. In the principal test conducted in Manchester, Edinburgh and Ulster simultaneously, the subjects being tested were not even institutionalised. No attempt was made to control their calories intake or to monitor the demands made in terms of calories expended. If ever any test was a travesty of science that one was.

The elements in a diet cannot be tested separately because they work as a team. Sometimes one does not work, unless another is present. This is true of the vitamins as well as polyunsaturated fats. This whole fallacious process of treating nutrients as if they were drugs is admirably explained by four leading American biochemists: Roger J Williams, James D Heffley, Man-Li-Yew and Charles W Bode in an article in *Perspectives in Biology and Medicine*, Volume 17, Number One, Autumn 1973.

Let me quote a short extract:

> The fourth basic fact in nutrition which has been sadly neglected by medical science is that of the essential "teamwork" among nutrients. Because this principle has been neglected, a whole unscientific concept has been widely accepted with respect to what a nutrient may be expected to do.
>
> This basic error, tacitly accepted, may be expressed as follows. Nutrients — amino acids, minerals and particularly vitamins — are potential "medicines" and should be tested accordingly, using statistical methods and suitable placebo controls to determine their efficiency in combatting diseases. If they prove to be specifics for particular diseases, well and good; if not, they must be regarded as medically worthless. In defence of this way of thinking is the historical fact that individual nutrients have in some cases acted like medicines — Thiamine, for beriberi, ascorbic acid for scurvy, niacinamide for pellagra. However, the parallel between these vitamins and medicines is more apparent than real, as careful consideration will show.
>
> Following this erroneous reasoning, it is concluded that, since specific individual nutrients are ineffective when

tested in this way against specific common ailments, these nutrients are worthless for combatting diseases. It is easy to conclude also that there should be no substantial concern regarding the intake of these nutrients on the part of the patients.

The joker in the argument is that, while no nutrient by itself is an effective remedy for any common disease, the nutrients acting as a team, are probably effective in the prevention of a host of diseases.

So much for the efforts of these American neurologists to establish that logic is as applicable in medical thinking as it is elsewhere. I return to my own efforts.

The principal reason to my mind, why research in neurology appears so fruitless, is because the problem being studied is not basically a medical problem but a biochemical one. I know that is a controversial statement, but please bear with me.

Try if you can to do what I asked you to do. Forget all you have been taught and think only of what can be logically and *pragmatically* demonstrated.

It can't, for instance, be proven that Multiple Sclerosis is a disease. That is an assumption and perhaps an unwarranted one. Professor Field claims to have proved it, but so far as I know his claim has not yet been generally accepted.

It has no obvious aetiology. No two are exactly alike. It is difficult to diagnose. Each case merges into all sorts of other closely related conditions.

There is one simple way of making sense of the confusion that surrounds all the degenerative diseases and that is to postulate that basically there is only one degenerative disease, that disease being tissue degeneration. It happens in an infinite variety of ways in every conceivable part, nook, cranny, organ, joint tissue of the human body. But always it is basically the same thing

— tissue degeneration.

Life is the constant renewal of cell tissue. Degenerative disease is the relentless breakdown of the same thing. Rather like some forms of death. Degenerative disease is in a sense the premature death of some part of the body. Degenerative diseases seem to be all familiar in their incidence though not directly hereditary. Thus there is clearly a genetic factor.

When I removed the following three substances from my diet — gluten, milk and sugar — two things struck me. First they were substances which caused a great deal of human misery in other ways. Gluten, for instance, is now held to be responsible for pernicious anaemia, certain liver complaints, sprue and other disabilities besides coeliac disease. Refined sugar causes diabetes, hypoglycaemia, dental caries and other problems. Milk, besides being bad for heart conditions, is increasingly being discovered to be responsible for many other ailments.

Why I wondered are these things bad for humans? Not why in the sense of what complex things are caused in the metabolism or in the cell tissue, because there I am not competent to observe. Why in the simple commonsense logical way.

When I looked for a possible reason, it wasn't long before it struck me that all three foods I had removed were comparative newcomers to the human diet — dating back several thousands of years at the earliest — from the time of the agricultural revolution when man ceased to be a hunter-gatherer and settled down to become a farmer.

Wheat was a mutation which occurred at that time in history, and made that revolution possible. Previously, wheat grass had a minute grain of 14 chromosomes. This crossed with goose grass which also had a tiny grain and the resulting plant had a fatter grain of 28 chromosomes. It happened to be fertile and there was another mutant which now had a reasonably fat grain of 42 chromosomes. This was the ancestor of our bread wheat. (My information in this matter comes from Dr Jacob Brunowski.) When man grew and ate this new food he was ingesting something which was not part of the normal diet on which the species had been developed over thousands of years.

Having settled as a farmer, man domesticated cattle, and cow's milk became a regular foodstuff. This too had never before been consumed regularly.

The same is true of sugar.

These three substances I had found reason to remove from my diet were all newcomers to mankind's diet, were all substances which had not over the ages of our existence been part of our normal diet.

This led to a new train of thought — the connection between an animal and the food it eats. A very simple example which occurred to me was the case of the silk moth. If the eggs of a silk moth are laid on any tree other than the mulberry, the silk worm will not survive.

In a sense the food and the living creature are different aspects of the same thing. The silk moth is the living form of the chemicals contained in mulberry leaf.

What about man?

Man is classified as omnivorous. But that is by no means to be understood as meaning that we can happily live on anything. Certainly we are not specialised in our eating habits, but it is my contention that we obey the same rule as do all other living creatures. This seems logical and it seems to offer an explanation for many otherwise inexplicable phenomena.

We are the living forms of the chemicals of the foods from which, over thousands of years, we have been created.

What is true of the silk worm, of the carnivore, of the

herbivore, must surely be equally true of man. His metabolism has been built from the chemicals in those foods from which over thousands of years he has been created.

What subtle differences or incompatibilities exist in these three new foods, I am obviously unqualified to judge. I submit that no one else is either. We would be incredibly arrogant to imagine that we know everything that is yet to be known about living matter. We would be equally arrogant to assume that man is unaffected by a phenomenon which appears to affect so many other creatures.

During the war many animals in London Zoo died because they were cut off from their normal foodstuffs and failed to thrive on apparently comparable substitutes. This information I got from someone who was a Fellow of the Royal Zoological Society at the time. It was this observation of his which first put me on to the idea that food intake is such a critical matter in the study of illness — a matter literally of life or death.

We must then make no arrogant assumptions about the breadth of our knowledge. All we can do is argue by analogy and act on pragmatically observed facts. Any neurologist's position, should he claim that he has to know in practical terms why my theory works before he will admit there may be something in it, would be a piece of unbelievably cruel and indefensible professional chauvinism. His position, were he to claim that he had proved that it does not work, by conducting a demonstrably inapplicable *medical* test on a biochemical phenomenon, would be equally unacceptable.

It is my contention that no neurologist is in a position to adopt either of these attitudes because his training has not covered the relevant areas. And yet I am sorry to have to say that I have encountered the attitude time and again.

The first neurologist with whom I began to discuss this theory dismissed me with the words "I don't know anything about biochemistry".

He was perfectly within his rights to say this. It was the simple truth. No one expected him to study biochemistry. But to me what he was saying might well have been: "I don't know anything about the cause of Multiple Sclerosis". And this again he would probably have to agree with. And if I added: "You're also saying that you don't know anything about the treatment of Multiple Sclerosis either", I'm afraid he would have to agree, because no treatment has yet been developed by the Establishment.

Only two relatively ineffective therapeutic treatments have been introduced. One is injection with Vitamin B12 and the other is the use of essential fatty acids, particularly in the form of the triglyceride esters of linoleic acid and gamma linoleic acid which are, I understand, the most complex molecules of these polyunsaturated fats yet discovered.

But if he put forward these as therapeutic treatments I would now agree with him. They are part of the therapy which I advocate. Why they have met with only minimal success when used by neurologists is, if I am right, because they are only two small parts of the complex jigsaw which has to be fitted together in order to control any individual case of the tissue degeneration known as Multiple Sclerosis in order to restore the patient's own cell building potential.

Also their success, in my estimation, depends on whether the individual being treated happens to suffer from a Vitamin B12 deficiency or from a particular weakness in his fat metabolism, or from some other problem.

I cannot stress too strongly my firm belief, founded both on theory and on my experience — remote though it is —

with more than twenty thousand sclerotics, that every case of Multiple Sclerosis is different from every other, that it is the way in which one particular individual's metabolism reacts to some particular imbalance in his diet when his genetic make-up to begin with contains a weakness in the nervous system.

It is my experience that there are three main groups of sclerotics connected with the three inimical foodstuffs I have identified. Because of the tendency of newspapers to encapsulate theories into brief headlines, my therapy has become known as the "gluten-free diet". This is totally inaccurate. In my opinion emphasis on the gluten-free aspect is no more, or less, important than the allergic reaction to sugar or to milk fat or to any other allergies which may be applicable, or to the other equally important factor, the deficiencies which can also be causative factors, for instance the deficiency in polyunsaturated fats, the deficiency in the B-group of vitamins — particularly perhaps B12 and other B vitamins like pantothenic acid, folic acid, thiamine and nicotinamide, and deficiencies in certain minerals — for example magnesium. From this brief list you can see how damaging and inadequate the press coverage has been on the reason for my success.

Not only is there a group of Multiple Sclerosis sufferers who react — sometimes almost immediately — to eating gluten, there is another group who tend towards and perhaps even suffer from diabetes or hypoglycaemia as well.

There is also a group who tend towards the illnesses connected with heart problems and I had a patient once whom I had walking with the aid of a cane and driving a car once more, who became bed-ridden again when her doctors forced her to remove only the B12 from my regimen. She resumed taking the B12 of course, and in a few months was driving again.

Neurologists in the main are scathing about my contention that gluten is connected with Multiple Sclerosis, more perhaps than about any of my other recommendations. And yet so far as I know no one knows exactly why it is that gluten has this harmful effect, in coeliac disease, on the mucosal lining of the bowel. It is known, from autopsies, exactly how it flattens out the actual lining, atrophies it, making it impervious to the nutrients which can no longer pass through it into the blood-stream. But it is not known why it does this. Until this is known it is perfectly logical for me to believe that gluten may have a similar damaging effect on mucosa or mucosal types of tissue anywhere else in the body. In sprue, for example, it causes some sort of ulcerous condition on the mucosal lining of the throat. Who is to say that it does not have a similar effect on comparable tissue elsewhere in the body — on the surface of the myelin sheaths in nervous diseases, on the tissue which separates brain and skull in Parkinson's disease, on the lining of the joints in arthritis?

As I keep repeating, the principles involved are not understood. We don't know why whales can achieve their enormous bulk by "eating" plankton and couldn't even assimilate a small sprat. We know something about it, and even more about the complex digestive processes needed to make protein out of wood in some herbivores and presumably in wood worms, but not enough is known yet for neurologists to take the hard-nosed stand they take in dismissing my theories which very few of them have even had the opportunity to study.

Not only is it possible that ingesting a number of harmful substances causes Multiple Sclerosis, it is becoming increasingly obvious to many people that the mistake, initiated thousands of years ago, by the agricultural revolution, is the reason for trouble all round.

Wherever you look in regimes intended to protect people from this or that degenerative trouble, you will find these three substances cropping up — bread, milk and sugar. They are selected purely pragmatically because of practical experience. So far as I know I am the first person to link them together into a viable rationale. I offer you a reason why it may be that these substances do so much damage in so many different ways. Why they are responsible for so many of the symptoms of those illnesses which are our greatest enemies, now that infections have been, to a great extent, controlled.

They produce the symptoms which doctors spend most of their time and effort in combatting. And yet many doctors today are themselves saying that it's wrong just to treat symptoms. What is the alternative? That is all that medicine is in one of its aspects — the treating of symptoms. One doctor published a statement recently in which he suggested that two thirds of the patients in hospitals at any one time were there recovering from the effects — the after-effects — of previous visits or of treatment by their General Practitioners. Again even if it is true, what is the alternative?

I suggest that the alternative is to go back beyond medicine. To go back to the very beginning of the subject, to go back to the simple fact of life. When the standard text-books on medicine were written in the nineteenth century — and before — no one really knew what life was. Now we know a little more. We know that it is a chemical process. Life itself is nothing but the constant renewal of cell tissue — a complex chemical process. And the chemicals involved are the chemicals of our food and drink. We are the living form of the chemicals we retain from what we eat and drink. The connection between us and the food we eat could hardly be more intimate.

Is it possible that the degenerative diseases are not

caused, as infectious diseases are, by some germ or virus attacking the body? Is it not possible — even likely — that they are caused by the breakdown of this elementary life process — caused by the body's inability to go on providing an adequate supply of healthy replacement tissue to the area involved?

Why might this happen? The answer is surely obvious. Our food intake is inadequate or wrong in some way. We are not ingesting the correct chemicals to allow our bodies to continue with their life function of producing adequate supplies of the multitude of different cells we require in order to remain healthy.

It's not just any old food we need. It's the food which contains those chemicals which, when put together in their living form, produce Homo Sapiens. We can't just live on grass as Nebuchadnezzar was alleged to have done. That only produces the life forms of herbivores. We can't live exclusively on plankton, though a whale can do that. We must live on those foods which man has been consuming since the beginning of his existence on earth — those foods of which man is the living counterpart. As you know, in my opinion these do not include cereals, sugar and milk.

Some people object that thousands of years is a long time and that by now we must have adapted to these foods. Let's consider this objection. What is the process of adaptation? It's the old Darwinian principle of survival of the fittest. Those who sicken and die obviously do not have progeny. But think of the degenerative diseases, for that is what we are talking about. Very few of them act before the reproductive phase of our lives has been successfully completed or at least begun. There is a very minimal loss in reproductive capacity in someone who succumbs to a degenerative disease.

In other words the mechanism of adaptation does not apply in the same way. We don't go through the Darwinian process of natural selection which would make our species adapt to these alien foodstuffs, and, as I've had occasion to say in another context, their effect is so slow that it is not easy to connect the degeneration they cause with their use.

What holds up therapeutic treatment in disease is that phrase of despair "Cause Unknown". It need no longer apply. The cause has remained unknown because researchers have been looking for it in the wrong place — among the effects. For the life of me, I can't see the logic behind this. Why expect to find the cause of a war by holding autopsies on the corpses on the battlefield or examining the damage caused to buildings? That method has led to such ridiculous suggestions as cell-senescence being put forward as the cause. Cell-senescence is very obviously the result, not the cause. The auto-immune syndrome seems to be similarly suspect.

A recent development in medicine seems to give further support to this possibility. The first crack seems to have appeared in this topsy-turvy scheme of researching the effects of an effort to find the cause. Dermatitis Herpetiformis has recently been explained by the acceptance of the fact that materials derived from food combine with immunoglobins (white blood cells, I take it) to form a substance which deposits in tissues and gives rise to illnesss.

Here we have a logic which could explain all degenerative conditions and justify my assertion that foodstuffs which are not the foods from which over the centuries we have been constructed, are alien to the human metabolism — as alien as are disease germs — and are rejected by our defence mechanisms, which, in their attempt to destroy this multitudinous invader leave wreckage around which damages the tissues they are trying to defend.

The whole auto-immunity syndrome is thus seen to be

quite possibly the effect and not cause — not cause of degeneration or "disease", but the result of eating the wrong foods. The auto-immune system, I suggest, is not in any way diseased or attacked by a virus. It is simply being overworked. If I am right, too, this new medical discovery could prove to help elucidate the cause not only of Dermatitis Herpetiformis, but of the whole spectrum of so-called diseases which are not those which can properly be called infectious.

Not only is the presence of a foodstuff which might be called an allergy, a possible cause of degeneration, it might be equally true that the absence of some substance could be a causative factor.

Structural fat, for instance, is necessary before cell tissue of any kind can be rebuilt. The body cannot begin to build one single cell unless structural fat is present. This fact which I have on the authority of a highly respected biochemist must account for a great deal of degenerative disease too.

Obviously when structural fat is absent the result will be the failure of the metabolism to build healthy normal cell tissue.

All that I have put forward in a general way about degenerative disease should obviously have some application to cancer, but that is such an emotive subject that I do not feel justified in putting forward theories or logical arguments either deductive or inductive which express my point of view. I would like however to quote from Elmer W Lammi of "United Press National" writing in the *Detroit News* of 30 July, 1976. "Dr Gio B Gori of the National Cancer Institute told a Senate Committee this week that recent experiments have raised the intriguing possibility of using nutrition as a direct form of cancer therapy".

And again, "Gori, deputy director of NCI's division of

cancer cause and prevention, said one major goal of current research is to determine the role of nutrition in the cause and prevention of cancer and disease in general".

Lastly, he said there was a "worldwide correlation between colon cancer and fat consumption", significantly one of the three foods I singled out for condemnation. I leave the reader to draw his own conclusions.

Blotches, blebs, sores, tumours, carbuncles, stiff joints, varicose veins, psoriasis all seem to me to be just lousy cell tissue created by a metabolism which, given the correct materials, has it in its power to create a healthy disease-free body.

And there is another obvious causative factor — the lack of essential minerals. If a certain mineral is necessary for the creation of a needed tissue and the metabolism doesn't have any available, that tissue just won't be made. Calcium for the manufacture of bone is a case in point, already recognised by everyone, and there must be many less obvious examples.

What I have outlined here is not a therapy but simply a principle. I have not claimed to know exactly what substances are needed to prevent the degeneration in every case, I have laid down a simple principle, namely that the failure of the metabolism to create healthy tissue is what causes degeneration.

I would like to go one step further and claim that no one will ever be able to lay down definitely what specific substances are required to treat any particular degenerative "diseases". The point here is that no two people necessarily have the same deficiencies or allergies which may be among the causative factors. Also, people live in different areas where different minerals may be lacking from either the water supply or the local foods.

What has to be faced is that every individual's degenerative disease is his own unique response to a

41

genetically inherited weakness. Having said this, however, it remains true that all degenerative conditions, in my opinion, have a large number of factors in common.

I think that every human being is damaged in the long run by ingesting the three foodstuffs I have singled out as our enemies. Some are more sensitive than others to one or other of them but it seems only common sense to believe that all of us are affected to some limited extent by all three.

The therapy which I developed to help my metabolism to rebuild its myelin sheath has to my certain knowledge helped many, many hundreds of others to do the same and has positively helped many, many others to rebuild other body tissues.

I am not claiming that I have developed a magical potion. What I have done is to rationalise a method of enabling the metabolism to resume its normal function of building healthy cell replacement tissue where the process has gone wrong.

The damage which has been caused by the erroneous belief that Multiple Sclerosis for instance is a "disease" is far-reaching and devastating. It leads people to think that it has the same cause in every case, that what helps one case, will help another. It has led to millions of pounds being wasted in research in the wrong direction — in an attempt to find the cause by analysing the effects.

Neurological thinking about Multiple Sclerosis seems to me to be not only misguided but misdirected. Even if a virus is discovered and a vaccine developed, it will simply delay the inevitable switch from symptom-treatment to cause-elimination. The vaccine-corrected sclerotic will still be vulnerable to attack by all other "diseases" from which he would be automatically protected if he took the simple precaution of filling his body only with the fuel on which over thousands of years it has been developed to run properly.

I'd like to finish if I may by putting forward the suggestion that medical thinking, in the area of the degenerative diseases, is an outworn paradigm, or system of rules, which will have to be replaced by a totally new point of view or scheme of practices, just as the Ptolemaic view of astronomy was gradually replaced by the new thinking of Copernicus, though this only came about slowly after fierce opposition from the sixteenth and seventeenth century establishments.

The Ptolemaic system seemed perfectly logical. Even today it still seems perfectly reasonable to postulate that the sun moves around the earth. Only a few highly specialised astronomers can disprove it. But it is now generally accepted that in fact the earth does move around the sun.

In the same way, the medical conception of degenerative diseases is an apparently logical proposition. Common sense appears to validate it. It just happens to be wrong. When Copernicus realised that the eccentric behaviour of the planets could be explained only by postulating that the earth and the planets moved round the sun, everything clicked into place. Inexplicable goings-on suddenly made sense.

It is exactly the same when you realise that degenerative conditions are not "diseases" — are not some strange germs or viruses attacking the body — but are, in fact, the chemical process of life itself going wrong, so that the body, instead of building healthy replacement cell tissue to keep itself in good repair, is lacking in the ingredients to do this and so fails to sustain good health. It is when you realise this, that everything puzzling and inexplicable in the field of degeneration suddenly clicks into place.

The overdrugging of the body for instance. Why use drugs against an enemy which isn't there? We only damage our own bodies when we should be nurturing them. We should be enabling the metabolism to build the needed replacement cell tissue. Instead of helping it, we are injuring it with lethal drugs, like the new chemo-therapy used in cancer and various forms of cortisone used by neurologists. Their use is justified only if there is no alternative. I suspect that the rationale I put forward provides one.

Then there is the medical obsession with symptoms. Why attack symptoms when you should be attacking the cause of the symptoms? The answer of course is that neurologists and other specialists in degenerative diseases have nothing else to attack because they don't know the causes. When I treated myself I left the symptoms severely alone and concentrated on restoring my metabolic health. In the result my symptoms vanished like snow in summer. In truth the symptoms of Multiple Sclerosis are not truly symptoms. The symptom is demyelination. Nystagmus, ataxia, tremor of intent, lack of balance, pins and needles, numbness and the rest are really secondary symptoms — effects of the demyelination.

Not only don't you have to attack these secondary symptoms, you don't have to attack the primary symptom either. No drug is needed to remove the damaged myelin tissue. What are needed are the nutrients which will enable the body to build healthy tissue to take its place. Infectious diseases, too, have clearly defined aetiologies. They respond in an identical way to the same therapy. If degenerative conditions *are* "diseases", why don't they behave in the same way? Obviously I would suggest because they are *not* "diseases".

As I see it, I have proved this point over and over again. But I need support, and I need help. I can't do it by myself. I think I have hit on the principle which governs the control of degeneration. I know certain of the factors which militate against the correct functioning of the metabolism, I've proved this by having a fantastic ratio of success to failure in the Multiple Sclerosis victims and others who do what I say strictly enough and for a long enough period. There is no way in which this can be an accidental lucky streak of always getting in touch with people who are about to have a remission. The last circular I sent out showed ninety per cent of people improving and sustaining their improvement.

It has to be admitted that I wrote to people who had already shown improvement — but even that is a vastly higher than 50% average. There seems to be little room for doubt that I have found the answer — but I need the help, not the opposition of the medical professions.

I am a layman, simply an intelligent victim who refused to accept despair as a viable way of life and was rewarded by the gift of renewed life and vigour.

Why do I appear to have succeeded where elaborate, expensive research has failed? I believe it is because I had no *medical* training and started without any preconceived ideas. When a researcher begins his work, he starts from a position which has been reached by his predecessors. He will only do valid research if the work of all those who went before him has been flawless.

Just as with a computer, faulty programming results in mistakes, so in any human endeavour undetected errors can persist for centuries and invalidate much of what follows.

The reception given at first to the ideas of Copernicus in astronomy, of Einstein or Plank in physics, Lister, Simpson, Pasteur and many others in medicine, of Darwin and Wallace in biology, of a whole list of innovators in fact, in many different fields, illustrates the point I am trying to make.

It is necessary for an Establishment to be conservative if

it is to guard against charlatans. Unfortunately, this unavoidably cautious outlook guards equally against innovators. Almost without exception in the course of history, new ideas have had to fight against old ones.

In the current approach to my own degenerative disease I have counted eleven assumptions which seem to me to be fallacious. I am sure I would find just as many in the, to me, unwarranted assumptions which doctors make before they begin to theorise about the other degenerative diseases.

In case any of you think I am exaggerating let me end by listing eleven fallacies.

The first and most dangerous fallacy is the unwarranted assumption that Multiple Sclerosis is a disease. In a sense the other fallacies follow from this simple mistake.

The second is the belief — encouraged by that first misconception — that it has one cause or group of causes in all cases.

The third is that what caused it in "A" will necessarily cause it in "B".

The fourth, that what helps "A" will necessarily help "B". These are just natural analogies mistakenly taken for granted because they appear to follow the first erroneous assumption. It follows, equally, inevitably, that doctors look on it as the sort of complaint for which a "cure" can be found as distinct from a "control" that, unlike coeliac disease and diabetes, for example, it is the sort of condition which is susceptible to cure. This is the fifth fallacy.

The sixth is the belief that it is contracted by the sufferer at a specific time or age whereas the truth would seem to be that one is born a sclerotic exactly as one is born a diabetic or a coeliac. Perhaps I should say a potential sclerotic, but I am sure you know what I mean.

The seventh fallacy is the assumption that it is a medical problem. I think I have made clear my belief that it is much more logically regarded as a biochemical and nutritional one.

The eighth is that neurologists believe that the "statistical probability" double blind trial with placebo is applicable where very obviously that can only apply to an experiment with only one variable factor.

The ninth is the one described by the American biochemists of failing to recognise the essential teamwork of nutrients and thinking they can be used in the same way as drugs.

The tenth I would claim to be the belief that drugs have any relevance in the treatment of Multiple Sclerosis — drugs, that is, whose purpose is to kill germs or bacteria. In Multiple Sclerosis it is my deep conviction that there is nothing there to be killed. What *is* there is an ailing metabolism crying out for the nutrients it needs in order to get on with the life-giving job of manufacturing a constant supply of healthy cell replacement tissue.

And now the last fallacious assumption that I mean to talk of tonight, although you can be sure it is not the last which will be unearthed when other minds more qualified than mine begin to see the truth of the principles upon which I have stumbled. This fallacy is the assumption that because the problem ends up in the nervous system, that is where it begins. As I said at the beginning, as logically assume that chickenpox or scarlet fever are problems for a dermatologist to deal with.

At various times tonight, I have generalised from my own specific experience and claimed that the principles that apply to my approach to Multiple Sclerosis apply equally to other degenerative diseases.

I would like to end by stressing this resemblance and underlining my belief that the fallacies I have spoken of in terms of the medical attitude to neurological conditions apply with equal force to the medical treatment of all

47

degenerative conditions.

Medicine in the degenerative diseases is a perfectly logical and acceptable system after a certain point. Beneath that point it is based on these fallacious assumptions which nullify the entire superstructure. The time has come for a new system to replace the fallacious substructure on the present one.

Medicine has to go back to square one, as I did in my totally self-motivated panic, and look on degeneration as a phenomenon much more closely allied to the natural process of death than to the medical realm of germ-caused diseases. You are born with the seeds of degeneration already there in your genetic inheritance. The trouble develops or is retarded according to the health or otherwise of what Claude Bernard called "the internal environment" — according, that is, to the effect of the nutrients you supply to your metabolic processes so that they can do the best possible job for you in building healthy replacement cell tissue for any areas which are susceptible to the slow death of degeneration.

3

Dietary Management

SHORTLY AFTER Roger MacDougall and I gave the lecture in the Netherlands two nuns approached us regarding dietary management. One of these nuns, who was in great form, had been following the Dr Evers diet for many years with good results. The other nun had started on the Roger MacDougall diet, also with good results. As the dietary regime of the one nun was totally different to the other's, it was quite understandable that these ladies wanted to question this.

Any dietary regime, and there are quite a few now, does change the Multiple Sclerosis patient some way or another. On the same programme some achieve better results than others, while some suffer a relapse. This last group of patients in particular should be under good guidance and control of a doctor or naturopath.

The question remains, however, why these diets all have an influence on Multiple Sclerosis patients. It is quite logical if we accept that one of the causes of Multiple Sclerosis is a defect in the metabolic system, we should also understand that a change to another form of diet can affect the condition of the patient very quickly. Mostly, the process of improvement is slow and all too often Multiple Sclerosis patients begin to lose heart after being on a certain programme for only a few months.

Multiple Sclerosis patients should realise that the disease, which has been developing very slowly, will disappear at an even slower rate and it will take time before any improvements can be expected. I often beg people not to give up, but to keep at it, because results can be expected in the long run.

The different diets followed by our two nuns were totally contradictory to each other. Yet, by the shock to the system through changing to a completely different diet, some way or another, remissions were reached. Both of these nuns have enjoyed a remission up until the time of writing, which shows that diet is most important and should be followed very strictly.

I have often stated that I am in favour of the Roger MacDougall diet, not only because basically it is very well balanced, but because it has cleared up other problems unconnected with Multiple Sclerosis. If followed strictly, there are no problems when it is supplemented with the necessary vitamins and minerals.

One should also keep a check on one's weight. If this should drop too low, it is necessary to include plenty of potatoes and nuts within this diet.

A Gluten-free diet on its own could be harmful, leading to vitamin and mineral deficiencies, so it is essential that the Multiples Sclerosis patient following the diet adheres to the instructions very carefully. Important points are:

1 no gluten
2 low sugars
3 low animal fats and high unsaturated fats

4 making good possible vitamin and mineral deficiencies

It is also most important to know which foods to avoid in this diet. The following summary gives an indication of these.

Gluten must be cut out rigidly. This means that one should avoid all use of wheat, barley, oats and rye, all of which contain gluten, and this also includes foods made from or containing these grains or the gluten from them, such as Weetabix, Shredded Wheat, Wheatgerm Flakes, Froment, All-Bran, white and brown bread, cakes, puddings, biscuits, porridge, rye and wheat crispbreads, all kinds of pasta, semolina, Bisto, etc. Eat nothing that has even a pinch of flour in it. In this respect your diet must be as strict as that of someone suffering from coeliac disease. In my opinion you would be wise to take this precaution even if gluten sensitivity is not yet apparent in your system.

Also, completely cut out all *refined sugar*. This is advice I would give to anyone whether or not sugar is shown to be an allergen. Nowadays, most medical authorities would agree on this. It is possible, however, that honey and fructose (fruit sugar) may be less damaging to your system.

One should severely limit the intake of *animal fats*. Cut out butter, cream and rich cheeses. Fresh milk should not be taken because it contains too much fat or cream, so use only skimmed milk, skimmed milk powder or goat's milk. Instead of butter, use margarine made from sunflower seeds, safflower seeds or corn oil.

Instead of olive oil, use sunflower or safflower seed oil for cooking and salads. (These oils deteriorate rapidly and should only be used once and thrown away.) Fried foods are the hardest to digest, so please try to reduce your intake.

Avoid all highly-saturated fats such as beef, pork, ham, goose, duck, mutton and lamb fats. Bacon, too, should be avoided. Whenever possible eat offal (liver, kidney, tongue, sweetbreads, etc.) in preference to meat. Eat free-range animals (venison, rabbit, poultry) in preference to domestic animals. Always remove the fat from your meat. In domestic animals the ratio of adipose (harmful) fat to structure (essential) fat can be 50 to one. In free-range animals it is 2 to one.

Beer, gin, whisky, vodka, sweetened fruit juices and bottled fizzy drinks are not permitted.

Although I consider the Roger MacDougall programme, as outlined before, a good dietary regime, I often point out to patients that, as the illness may be due to allergies and deficiencies, they should undergo extensive allergy tests. After the allergy-testing I may change the diet to suit the individual's needs. Changing the diet to eliminate the patient's most common allergies, a good bio-chemical balance may be achieved, thus relieving the symptoms. Again it is of vital importance that the removal of certain foods should be compensated by the correct vitamin, mineral and trace element supplements.

Geographically, it is most interesting to see (from several studies) why in countries like The Netherlands, Belgium, Germany, Scandinavia and The United States of America the incidence of Multiple Sclerosis is so much higher than in southern countries. It is almost accepted, as shown again in many studies, that it depends on how fats are broken down by the individual processes and that the ability to handle these fats is connected with a deficiency in the essential fatty acids.

We certainly all agree, especially in Scotland, that diet is of vital importance, not only in the cause, but also in the treatment of Multiple Sclerosis. Fat consumption in the Scottish diet is one of the highest in the world. Hospital admissions for alcoholism in Scotland are seven times higher than in the rest of the United Kingdom, while bowel cancer occurrence in Scotland is 90% higher than in the rest of the UK. Incidence of cancer generally is the second highest in the world, while deaths from strokes have been the highest in the world.

These are just a few figures given in the excellent book *The Health Revolution* written by Ross Horne, which really makes us think. In my mind there is no doubt that diet plays a large role in this.

Although many diets are used in the approach to Multiple Sclerosis, they all have some common factor, such as the use of plenty of fresh fruit and vegetables, nuts, seeds, seed-oils; no refined foods; care with additives; no smoking; preferably no alcohol; very little or no saturated fats.

Disagreement exists over the use of meat, sugar, dairy products and gluten in grains.

This briefly outlines some basic rules in diets which are designed for Multiple Sclerosis patients.

When I have successfully identified a food allergy, it always gives me pleasure to see the patient improve when the food is cut out. Often, Multiple Sclerosis patients question their ability to stick to the new diet. But what is the alternative? Continued deterioration. It may take time — but it's worth it. Roger MacDougall stuck to his diet for four years before his frozen fingers, one glorious day, managed to do up a shirt button. All the encouragement he had was a burning conviction that his reasoning was sound and the fact that after a while he stopped deteriorating. So I say once more: hold on and continue until physical improvements can be noticed. He, after all, was starting from rock bottom — total paralysis and lack of balance and almost complete loss of speech and sight.

I have said before that it is important to take

supplements and in the next chapter I will go into this in more detail.

The following letter shows for itself how rewarding it is when people keep strictly to the instructions of the diet:

One year has passed since the start of my treatment with you and I felt the time was opportune to tell you of my gratitude. In my eyes the task which you set yourself was enormous but I am glad to say, the effort was most certainly worthwhile. But how can I thank you enough in the most appropriate terms?

The only way I feel able to do so, is to remember how the years have affected me and how within the last year alone I have made the most remarkable recovery.

I recall that as the years have passed how my walking ability diminished; developing bladder trouble; defective eyesight; depressions; bad temper; slurred speech and waning interest.

When I met you on 7 September 1974, I had already been on the gluten free diet (which incidentally still included "sugar" or sucrose) and at that time my condition was holding its own against further deterioration. After my first consultation I realised that I had no option but to rigidly adhere to the stricter diet you gave me. At that same meeting you introduced me to the ancient treatment of Acupuncture.

Since that meeting my life has changed from the mumbling, crumbling existence to one of renewed vigour and confidence. All the ailments have cleared or are beginning to improve. The evidence I present must surely speak for itself.

The day cannot be far away when I am able to battle with the golf courses I played on when "fit". What a change indeed!

I do, as you know, hold a position of significance in Scotland and I can now give this position attention of a more concentrated and vigorous nature which should be mutually rewarding.

4

Vitamins, Minerals and Trace Elements

IT IS important to know that people following a diet and cutting out certain foods can deprive themselves of beneficial vitamins, minerals and trace elements, the shortage of which could be harmful. When gluten is being dropped from the diet a definite substitute of certain vitamins is needed. Omitting milk could be harmful because of its animal fat content. In addition, it is a source of Vitamins B2, B12 and Calcium.

The best way of course is to eat other foods which contain these vital substances. However, one has to be very careful and as it is important for every Multiple Sclerosis patient to use certain vitamins, I would advise a supplement. In line with the Roger MacDougall programme a very good formula was developed, which is as follows:

Choline Bitartrate	10.0 mg
Vitamin B1	2.0 mg
Vitamin B2	1.0 mg
Vitamin B6	6.0 mg

Vitamin C	25.0 mg
Vitamin E	7.5 mg
Folic Acid	0.015 mg
Inositol	10.0 mg
Nicotinamide	40.0 mg
Calcium-D-Pantothenate	12.0 mg
Calcium Glutonate	75.0 mg
Magnesium Carbonate	75.0 mg
Lecithin	25.0 mg

This formula is an important supplement in the treatment of Multiple Sclerosis, but these tablets and capsules should not, as is sometimes indicated, be seen as a cure for Multiple Sclerosis. They are a safeguard to supplement the altered diet, but many people feel that they give them a good source of energy.

The best way of course to supplement basic shortages of these vitamins is to take plenty of fresh food, fresh vegetables, natural foods and to balance all this, a good intake of rice. Rice is an excellent remedy, called the yin and yang food in China. Here is a very good recipe.

Put whole brown rice in a casserole or a pyrex dish. Pour boiling water over the rice and place the dish in a preheated oven. Cook it for 10 to 15 minutes and switch off the heat. Keep rice in the oven for 5 to 6 hours. Cut up some vegetables such as parsley, chicory, celery and cress and mix this through the rice with a little garlic salt. Heat it up and the rice will be ready for use.

Do not underestimate the importance of a good balanced diet. Although these vitamins specified are made of 100% biological natural ingredients and manufactured under strictly controlled conditions, it is nevertheless important that a healthy diet is taken care of.

As I have said before, one should see every Multiple Sclerosis patient as a completely individual case.

There is growing evidence in the United States that Multiple Sclerosis might be related to a virus, or to an allergy or even perhaps to an inherited problem. It is also known that if the cause were due to a virus, that virus remains in the wall of the small intestine. One of its products is super oxide radical. This radical is responsible for the destruction of the myelin sheath. The treatment plan based on this hypothesis is threefold.

First the virus must be removed from the body. This will be accomplished by using Interferon stimulance and immunoglobulins. Secondly the super oxide radical must be removed, utilising the dismutation reaction. Thirdly the physiological condition of the organ systems of the body must be restored to an optimum level.

Dr Harold Manner from the United States, with whom I work closely, has developed a schedule to be used in his clinics, which was printed for the practising physician. Added to this, however, was the warning that it should in no way be considered as a do-it-yourself manual. Professional diagnoses and regular checks are absolutely essential to the success of the treatment on this programme.

Vitamin and mineral levels of the Multiple Sclerosis patient are usually out of balance — it is therefore essential that the body be brought back to normal as rapidly as possible. Once vitamin and mineral deficiencies and surpluses are known, measures can be taken to correct the imbalance.

Although we know that all the Vitamin B complex is important to the Multiple Sclerosis patient, we should realise that Vitamin C is also of great importance. I have often come across improvement in the condition of Multiple Sclerosis patients after using Interferon. As this is sometimes difficult to obtain, we should remember that its production can be stimulated by Vitamin C. Hence the conclusion that a high dosage of Vitamin C for the Multiple Sclerosis patient can sometimes be beneficial.

By a dismutation reaction, the super oxide radical reacts with hydrogen under the influence of super oxide dismutase to produce hydrogen peroxide. This peroxide is then converted to water and pure oxygen under the influence of either peroxidase or catalase. This can be accomplished in the body by using dismutase tablets. However, I have found that using the mineral Germanium, which gives a boost release of oxygen, has been of great benefit to Multiple Sclerosis patients.

It is also important to stimulate the immune system. One can give Vitamin A in an emulsified form, which increases the number of circulating lymphocytes. Lymphocytes are additionally stimulated by the addition of thymosine, which will also help the immune system of a Multiple Sclerosis patient.

Vitamin E is essential to prevent oxidation of unsaturated fats and is also advised to be taken when on a gluten-free diet which excludes wheatgerm. Sometimes we advise patients to add a little extra Vitamin E to the amount which is recommended in the Roger MacDougall programme.

Vitamin F is also essential and is found in Oil of Evening Primrose, which is dealt with in a later chapter. When using Oil of Evening Primrose it is of great importance that cod-liver-oil or a good fish oil is used to link up with this particular treatment.

One of the most important minerals for the Multiple Sclerosis patient is Zinc. Some Multiple Sclerosis patients, who have a tendency to get depressed and downhearted, often benefit from additional Zinc. This mineral has the exceptional property of boosting the patient's morale when depression occurs.

Futhermore we have Copper, Iron, Magnesium and

Selenium — all of which minerals are found helpful in the total treatment of Multiple Sclerosis. Another much newer report is on Lecitone which is a migration of lipid complexes in the body.

In order to better understand the efficacy of a dietary supplement based on dehydrated brain rich in brain lipid complexes, their migration in the body should be studied. This has been carried out more particularly with phospholipids which represent the essential of lipid complexes of the brain.

Mention must be made firstly of a publication of Gregoriadis who, in 1977, in Life Sciences, presented a remarkable summary of the biological role of lipid complexes. He noted that phospholipids are the essential constituants of intracellular biological membranes and that they are arranged in molecular layers characterised by a semi-liquid crystalline state. This physico-chemical characteristic being dependent upon the length and degree of unsaturation of the fatty acid chains, Gregoriadis emphasises the fragility of such membranes and the movements of phospholipid molecules. He explains phospholipid transfers occurring within a particular membrane, from one membrane to another and diffusions of exogenous phospholipids which are exchanged with damaged molecules. These findings led to the following conclusion: this dynamic state of phospholipids within or across cellular membranes as well as between cellular organelles is very relevant not only to the possibility of intercellular exchange of phospholipids but also to the mechanism of utilisation of exogenous phospholipids.

1. *Lipid complexes and the intestinal barrier.*
In 1948, C Artom and A Swanson reported that phospholipids must play a role in the absorption of fatty acids, and envisaged the possibility of absorption of intact

phospholipid molecules through the intestinal barrier: one cannot dismiss the possibility of a direct absorption of intact phospholipids, a possibility which is also suggested by the ease with which the compounds are emulsified in water.

The first study carried out under strict conditions with synthetic phospholipids labelled with C^{14} and P^{32} was published in 1955 by Blomstand, who was able to show that a notable proportion of ingested phospholipids were found in the lymph.

In 1947, Robert Scow and Y Stein used labelled soya lecithin, showed that 40% of phospholipids present in the chylomicron were of dietary origin. They also showed that lecithin was absorbed in the form of lysolecithin, immediately reacylated in the intestine: the findings indicate that dietary lecithin is hydrolysed and absorbed as lysolecithin and subsequently reacylated before being incorporated into lymph chylomicrons.

More recently, administering small amounts (2.3 mg/kg) of *labelled synthetic lecithin* per os in the dog, K Schmid concluded: "in the dog the drug is totally and rapidly absorbed, while the elimination of the radioactivity is very slow". In fact, the first traces of lecithin are found in the blood after one hour, the level is maximum after 24 hours and remains high seven days later.

The same author showed in the rat that the distribution of lecithin administered orally or intravenously was virtually uniform in the principal tissues, including the brain.

— The study of D Lekim and E Graf published in 1976 and involving *double labelled soya phospholipids* with high doses (70 mg/kg per os in the rat) reach the same conclusion: the absorbed radioactivity rose up to 90%, 24 hours after oral applications of 70 mg/kg. The absorbed radioactivity was incorporated into all organs but to quantitatively different degrees. These authors confirm that phospholipids are converted to lyso derivatives and immediately reacylated.

2. *Lipid complexes and the blood-brain barrier.*
After having reviewed the principal studies showing the passage of phospholipids through the intestinal barrier, it is important to study their migration through the body and in particular to the brain.

—in 1972 le Kim reported a study using *double labelled synthetic lecithin administered intravenously* in the rat and studied their migration into tissue cells. He showed that blood phospholipids were taken up intact by the cells, leading to the following conclusion: All these results together compile sufficient evidence for an entrance of complete lecithin molecules into eucaryot cells and their association with cellular structures such as mitochondria and miscrosomal membranes.

—In 1969 Hoelzl and Franck published a study concerning the passage of phospholipids into the brain. They used a double labelled phosphatidylcholine to demonstrate that there is no blood-brain barrier for phospholipids.

—In 1971, G B Ansell wrote as follows: that the phosphatidylcholine in the brain comes unchanged from the liver by way of the blood is therefore a possibility. Amongst other findings the author reported that choline reached the brain in the form of lecithin: It seems almost certain that choline is supplied to the brain by the blood in a lipid-bound form as either phosphatidylcholine or as its lysoderivative.

—In a publication dating from 1972, R Illinworth and

O Portman noted that lysolecithins accounted for 5-20% of plasma phospholipids. They studied their role by injecting monkeys with a *labelled synthetic lysolecithin* and were able to demonstrate that it was taken up and metabolised by the brain where it acted as a precursor for lecithin and choline. Lysolecithin thus appeared to be the transporter of choline to the brain since: "Adult brain is unable to synthetise choline *de novo*". The most remarkable finding in this study was demonstration that the conversion of lysolecithin to lecithin occurs in a specific manner for the brain since the lecithin formed is characteristic. This is one of the first occasions of the demonstration of organ specificity for phospholipids: our findings that the relative specific radioactivities of tetraenoic phosphatidylcholine species from brain were two to three times as great as those of other fractions are consistent with current views on phosphatidyl choline biosynthesis.

Working with double labelled *phospholipids extracted from the brain*, P Orlando studied the kinetics of cerebral phospholipids. Administration by injection and per os of 100 mg/kg of cerebral phospholipids led to the following conclusion: we show that brain phospholipids, administered to animals can cross the blood barrier unaltered, and remain stable in the brain so long as to exhibit their peculiar pharmacological effects . . . the results suggest that there is a continuous passage of the phospholipids from blood to brain, with a replacement of the hydrolysed molecules.

This latter remark is important since it shows that exogenous phospholipids may replace damaged membrane phospholipids.

3. *Are cerebral phospholipids specific?*

It is known that certain tissues are highly specific with regard to their lipid composition. This is the case in particular of nerve or retinal cells which contain highly unsaturated phospholipids. Under such circumstances, it would be reasonable to anticipate specific uptake of exogenous lipids extracted from homologous sources.

Thus in 1961, W Schlemmer published a study demonstrating organ specificity with exogenous phospholipids extracted from the heart.

It has already been mentioned earlier that, in a 1972 publication, O Portmann showed that the synthesis of cerebral phospholipids was orientated towards a characteristic type of fatty acids.

In 1971, R Infante made an interesting comparison between the absorption of double labelled phospholipids extracted from liver and extracted from brain. The results showed that the uptake of brain phospholipids in the brain was much greater than that seen after the administration of hepatic phospholipids, leading the author to state: "Comparison of the uptake of hepatic and cerebral phospholipids in the two organs showed a marked preferential distribution in the organ from which the preparation has been made. This preferential uptake is not due to chance. Considering on the one hand the high level of transhepatic blood flow in comparison with that of the brain, and secondly the ease of blood-cellular exchanges in the hepatic cells in comparison with cerebral cells, it would seem to be obvious that the tropism of cerebral phospholipids by nerve cells corresponds to an active physiological mechanism, the nature of which remains to be elucidated."

> —More recent data are of obvious interest with regard to a possible specific phospholipid-tissue interaction. For example, A Bruni and G Toffano

have shown that alone amongst several phospholipids of different origin, phosphatidyl-serine extracted from bovine brain was capable of causing an increase in blood glucose after injection.

—Finally, I wish to mention the studies of P Orlando and G Porcellati published in 1976. These authors first worked *in vitro* and showed that lecithin or lysolecithin stimulated the synthesis of phospholipids. It should be noted that this stimulation occurs by a direct action on phosphorylcholine cytidyltransferase, the action of which was approximately tripled, regardless of the origin of the lecithin used (synthetic, extract from egg or from a tissue of some sort).

Continuing their investigation, the same authors studied *in vivo* the biosynthesis of brain phospholipids. They noted that egg lecithin or lysolecithin had no stimulating action on the *de novo* formation of phospholipids, but, on the contrary, clearly demonstrated that the lecithin extracted from bovine brain had a slight stimulating action.

These results demonstrate within the brain a specificity of activity of phospholipids on the organs from which they are derived.

They also imply that the administration of exogenous lipid complexes not only have a replacement action but will also play a regulatory role on the biosynthesis of endogenous lipid complexes (phospholipids).

5 *Conclusions*

Phosphorylated lipid complexes bound to highly polyunsaturated fatty acids form the basis of the biological membranes which control neurone metabolism. These brain lipid complexes have specific chemical character-istics.

The biological membranes are extremely fragile and may undergo disturbances in their physicochemical characteristics. Thus the saturation of double bonds or interruption of the elongation of fatty acids chains results in disturbances in the function of the human brain.

A dietetic preparation based upon dehydrated brain and vitamin E with its protective effect against oxidation of double bonds is capable of providing nerve cells with essential factors in the protection of their integrity.

Animal or tissue culture studies have shown that exogenous intake of brain lipid complexes have a specific action in favourising myelinisation and protecting nerve cells.

Several studies have also shown that brain phosphorylated lipid complexes administered per os cross the intestinal barrier and migrate preferentially to the brain.

All of these findings taken together justify the definition of the preparation LECITONE: food for the nerves.

The activity of this dietetic preparation has been confirmed clinically in the child suffering from fatigue during growth and in the adult with fatigue.

It is really not too difficult to find out what each individual's metabolic problem might be. It could be allergies or vitamin/mineral deficiencies or a faulty immune system. One common factor, however, is that the immune system must be boosted as much as possible.

Both my friends and colleagues, Dr Harold Manner and Professor Roger MacDougall, agree that the Multiple Sclerosis patient does not really suffer from a disease. It is more like suffering from an individual or unique imbalance which has its own specific cause. It is our responsibility to deal with this in a positive manner. It is no use to sit down and say: "I've got a problem and I've got to live with it". The condition must be treated as a challenge, knowing that if a positive approach is taken, then the goal will be reached.

5

Oil of Evening Primrose

EVENING PRIMROSE is a little plant with bright yellow flowers which originated in North America. In the olden days Indians used it for medicinal purposes. It has been known for a long time that the extract of this little plant has great healing powers for skin conditions and is beneficial to the healing of infections.

Recently this plant has created a lot of interest. It was noticed that people who were using an extract from this plant healed more quickly after an operation than people who were not using it. Later, researchers looked into possible benefits for arthritis, skin and menopausal problems. Of course in the present context my main interest is in their findings relating to Multiple Sclerosis.

One might expect it to be a complex matter to find out exactly why the extract is beneficial but it contains one very important molecule, the gamma linoleic acid, or GLA as it is sometimes called, which is essential for health.

Many people have difficulty in converting linoleic acid into GLA. Oil of Evening Primrose has proven its value in providing people with health benefits which they otherwise would not possess. Most important is the conversion of linoleic acid into GLA. Until GLA is produced it cannot be turned into the fatty acids which are vital to our health.

Linoleic acid is a polyunsaturate and one of the most important substances in our food. This essential fatty acid, like vitamins, is necessary in the maintenance of a healthy body.

Most scientists have now come to the conclusion that linoleic acid plays a significant role in the prevention of all kinds of degenerative illnesses as well as heart diseases. Because of this they realise the importance of Oil of Evening Primrose.

In this day and age there are many reasons why people get a deficiency of GLA. Convenience foods, hard margarine, certain biscuits and products which are high in saturated fats such as butter, milk or red meat, can hinder the production of GLA in some individuals. It is also an accepted fact that serious illnesses, including cancer, can be caused by over-indulgence in alcohol. This creates deficiencies of several elements which cause the body to stop producing GLA.

In order to get the best benefit from Oil of Evening Primrose, researchers have found over the years that combining this oil with other vitamins and minerals enhances the health of the individual.

With a GLA content of 9%, Oil of Evening Primrose is by far our richest source of this nutrient. Because this natural product can be used as a dietary supplement there is no problem of using drugs. It does not force the body to do or produce anything, but as shown in recent research and tests by several scientists, it is almost unbelievable what this little yellow plant is capable of. Maybe not for every patient, but certainly for many, the improvements have been dramatic and it would be worthwhile to prescribe this extract, on trial for a lengthy period of time, to every Multiple Sclerosis patient.

In 1979 four hundred and eighty Multiple Sclerosis sufferers took part in a particular survey while using Oil of Evening Primrose and it is hopeful to learn that of the participants 65% felt there was some improvement in their condition. Of these:

— 43% thought there was a stabilisation in their condition;

— 22% said they had suffered less severe attacks;

— 20% felt an alleviation of particular problems;

— 13% felt an improvement in their general health, and

— 2% reported further beneficial side-effects.

The full results were:

some improvement	65%
no change	22%
deteriorated	10%
don't know	3%

On my most recent visit to South Africa last year, I interviewed quite a number of Multiple Sclerosis sufferers. Where Oil of Evening Primrose was used in combination with certain fish oils, a large majority reported surprising results.

During his research my friend, Dr Hassam, found a shift in the proportion of saturated and unsaturated fatty acids recorded in the brains of Multiple Sclerosis patients. This was not totally unexpected, although results were inconsistent. This is often the result of a metabolic or nutritional disturbance during the period of brain growth, rather than during adulthood. Therefore it is most important that nutrition, as discussed before, be taken into consideration while using remedies like Oil of Evening Primrose.

Luckily, taking these measures, a remission may be long standing or permanent. Of the various methods which are being used nowadays, this one seems to be most successful.

Unfortunately the EFA — Essential Fatty Acids — are often ignored. One should never forget that fat is present in every cell of our body and that roughly 60% of the structure of the brain is composed of fat. EFA is vital for the proper growth and development of the brain as well as the total nervous system.

In Multiple Sclerosis cases the whole central nervous system is under attack. An unusual pattern of fatty acids has shown up in Multiple Sclerosis sufferers. By taking a diet rich in EFA it was demonstrated that this pattern can be reversed within the period of one year. Even back in the seventies it was discovered that relapses were less frequent and that great successes were achieved in the rebuilding of the immune system when using sunflower-oil.

Several laboratories have confirmed that Multiple Sclerosis patients have a low concentration of Essential Fatty Acids, plasma, red blood cells and platelets in the nervous system.

To investigate this a co-ordinated double-trial, lasting two years, was set up in Belfast and in London. The diets of the Multiple Sclerosis patients were supplemented with either sunflower-oil or olive-oil and at the end of the trial it was found that relapses tended to be less frequent and that a better control was achieved by those on sunflower-oil.

Professor Fields reached objective conclusions in his work and survey of Multiple Sclerosis. Further research is showing excellent results and will prove beneficial in the management of Multiple Sclerosis.

The dosage for Oil of Evening Primrose is variable. Personally I prescribe four to six capsules per day. They are easily taken, and sometimes my advice is to gradually build up the dosage. Do not give up too quickly, but persevere as it may take some time before effects are noticeable. People are often critical but once they are interviewed one discovers that they have only been using this extract for a short period of time.

A good capsule should contain not only Oil of Evening Primrose but also marine oil, so that with these two biologically active fatty acids the right supplement is administered.

Occasionally I have prescribed a higher dosage than normal, especially where I felt it desirable to speed up the process. Once I had a patient who told me why she really needed to see some improvement within the span of one year. I will end this chapter by telling you her story.

This patient was unable to walk and spent her life in a wheelchair. For some reason she came to me convinced that I would be able to cure her overnight. I had to tell her that it is impossible to cure Multiple Sclerosis, but that it might be possible to control it.

I discovered that she had four sons, two of whom intended marrying the following year. I could not fail to notice the anxious look in her eyes when she told me that she wanted to walk out on that day, even if it was just in and out of the church. She assured me that she would do anything to achieve this.

I told her that I would treat her to the best of my ability and felt that a high dosage of Oil of Evening Primrose might show some results. She followed my instructions to the letter and after some months she was able to cross the street in Glasgow where she lived, without any assistance. She did this much to the surprise of the policeman who was regularly on traffic duty there. He actually left his post for a moment to enquire what caused the improvement.

Mentally, this lady had been totally convinced that her condition could be improved, and she was committed to do anything within her power to help herself. She followed strictly and adhered to all the instructions given to her, but I still believe that the Oil of Evening Primrose was a great boost in this case.

I would recommend Multiple Sclerosis sufferers to try Oil of Evening Primrose as I have seen many cases in which it has been beneficial.

6

Hyperbaric Oxygen

SOMETIME DURING the evening, after lecturing on Multiple Sclerosis in 1975 in Bienne, Switzerland, I was approached by Professor Dr Karl Asai from Japan, who has done a lot of research into the mineral Germanium. We had a very worthwhile conversation which continued well into the night.

Professor Asai has done much research on cancer patients, but he also noticed that Germanium had a good influence on those suffering from Multiple Sclerosis. One of the characteristics of the mineral Germanium is that it releases a lot of oxygen. Bearing this in mind, I have treated several patients with this mineral whenever I have been able to obtain it (as the process used to make it soluble is very intricate).

Almost miraculous results were obtained when I treated a Dutch patient of mine. I still doubt, however, that the diagnosis of Multiple Sclerosis in this patient was correct as she only displayed some symptoms peculiar to Multiple Sclerosis and no lumbar puncture was performed on her. Nevertheless the fact remains that Multiple Sclerosis patients do react positively to Germanium. Consequently, when hyperbaric oxygen tests were established in Scotland, I followed their findings with added interest. I decided to try Germanium on some patients, who came to me after having had several treatments in an oxygen chamber. Positive results showed in improvements of double vision, speech and bladder control.

During this test period I was fortunate to meet Dr Ray Evers from the United States of America who has used a hyperbaric oxygen chamber in his clinic for many years. He told me that he once read an article entitled "Is oxygen the missing piece in the ageing process and its related health problems?" The article stated that even though water, juices, green juices and pure foods cleanse the body, unless there is an adequate supply of oxygen we have no solid foundation for life. A lack of oxygen in the system will prevent oxidation, which energises cells into a biological regeneration. The healing powers of oxygen have long been known. However, until the advent of hyperbaric oxygen — HBO — therapy, scientists were unable to uniformly introduce pure oxygen into the body's tissues.

Dr Evers began hyperbaric oxygen treatment in his health centre in Cottonwood, Alabama, in 1981. He found it an effective adjunctive therapy in the treatment of chronically degenerative diseased patients. He also told me that patients feel well after the treatment and that he did not discover any side-effects. Treatment in a hyperbaric oxygen chamber is pleasant enough, but should always be administered by trained people.

Research has shown hyperbaric oxygen therapy to be an effective treatment not only for Multiple Sclerosis, but also for people with other chronic degenerative diseases.

It depends totally on the patient how often treatments should take place. It is also very important that the atmospheric pressure to which the patient is subjected is carefully researched.

Under normal circumstances oxygen is transported by haemoglobin, carried in the red blood cells. These cells are usually 98% saturated with oxygen. However the red cells constitute only about 45% of the blood volume. Another carrier of O_2 is blood plasma. When the hyperbaric pressure is increased to two or more times the normal atmospheric pressure, the plasma becomes oxygen-rich to as much as ten to fifteen times its normal level. In fact the plasma of patients receives enough oxygen to sustain life for a considerable period of time.

Dr Ray Evers also said that he did not claim hyperbaric oxygen treatment as a panacea for all chronic degenerative diseases. He has however seen dramatic results in many chronically degenerated patients who demonstrated oxygen deprivation. The guideline in the treatment of everything, from cancer to gangrene, is that the body is starved of oxygen, suffers poor circulation and is the unwilling victim of induced poisons and poor nutrition.

I am aware that Dr Evers has done a lot of valuable research over the years and for that reason I advised my patients to get in touch with the ARMS organisation for the treatment of hyperbaric oxygen now available in this country.

In an article written by Dr James from the Watson Institute, Dundee University, I read that several ARMS centres have now been operative for over a year and many patients have been able to benefit from oxygen therapy. However it also seems that patients and their families are confused about any relationship between the cause of Multiple Sclerosis and the use of hyperbaric oxygen.

Dr James states very clearly that Multiple Sclerosis is often described as a demyelinating disorder in which the myelin sheaths are separated from the nerve fibres. It is possible that some myelin sheaths may be reformed, although the evidence to date is that nerve fibres cannot be replaced. Often the myelin sheath acts as an insulator. In fact the myelin sheath is present to increase the speed of conduction of the nerve impulse along the fibre.

Some of the facts show cause for optimism as it is proven that fat embolism can produce plaques in the human brain. These plaques are identical to those seen in established Multiple Sclerosis patients.

Patients known to have suffered from acute fat embolism can deteriorate in the same progressive way as Multiple Sclerosis patients. Fat embolism may therefore be one cause of Multiple Sclerosis, but it remains to be seen if it actually is the cause.

The clinical features of Multiple Sclerosis are entirely compatible with fat micro embolisms. Proof that the basic pathology in most Multiple Sclerosis patients is due to fat embolism is difficult to provide, although there is massive circumstantial evidence.

It is therefore most important for everyone to realise that the use of hyperbaric oxygen in treatment does not require this proof, because the pathological features already established indicate that it is an agent of choice. Dr James came to these conclusions after excellent investigation on hyperbaric oxygen treatment. One of the most interesting things I read in this particular paper was that most drug treatments used for symptomatic therapy cause significant side-effects. Oxygen is simply restoring the most favourable conditions for natural recovery.

In a world-wide test about 3000 Multiple Sclerosis patients were treated with hyperbaric oxygen, and the controlled studies proved its efficacy. Considerable improvement was obtained after exposure to HBO treatment — significant enough to carry on further testing.

A vital key for long life is that we carry an adequate

supply of oxygen in our bloodstream. A continuous supply of oxygen is necessary to our survival and today with constant atmospheric interference, it is important that we try to get out in the fresh air, sea air or mountain air, anywhere to get away from gases which are poisonous and to fill our lungs with oxygen.

Our brains require oxygen to function properly, giving us more mental activity. We should never forget that the air consists of a mixture of 21% oxygen, 78% nitrogen and minor traces of other gases.

There are approximately 60 trillion cells in the human body and each cell is responsible for hundreds of chemical reactions to support life and requires the correct amount of nutrients and adequate oxygen. If the circulatory system is obstructed many of these cells will starve from lack of oxygen, become diseased and will eventually die.

Breathing oxygen in cases of Multiple Sclerosis can sometimes affect improvement, but if the oxygen transport system is not functioning properly, hyperbaric oxygen treatment, in combination with Germanium, can improve the condition of a patient beyond belief.

The liver, which has to cope with influences from a variety of food and drink, suffers if its ally, oxygen, is not supplied in sufficient quantities to aid it with its intricate laboratory work.

With many Multiple Sclerosis patients I have paid extra attention to the liver. This was mostly done with the help of some liver-cleansing products and in a later chapter I will discuss some natural remedies which help the liver in its complicated work.

I constantly remind Multiple Sclerosis patients of the bad influence of alcohol and smoking, which really prevents them from improving their condition. Using Kirlian photography and comparing photographs which are taken before treatment, with those taken after the diet is altered and smoking and drinking is cut down or out, significant differences are noticeable. One can see that the oxygen transport system is once more working normally.

It is important that Multiple Sclerosis patients take plenty of exercise and in particular do good breathing exercises to aid the transport of oxygen. Glycogen is a great source of energy but it is limited by the amount of O_2 present. Oxygen therefore becomes a limiting factor so it is important that enough is present for the effective use of glycogen.

Relaxation exercises in any form, especially when the Multiple Sclerosis patient is under stress, will always increase oxygen to the tissue cells. A decrease of oxygen will lead to the unavailability of oxygen to the lymphocytes, which in turn will upset the hormonal balance supply of oxygen in the body.

Lymphocytes are normally contained in blood vessels. They leave the blood vessels to maintain the immunological balance of the body. Multiple Sclerosis patients lack oxygen and this decreases the ability in the brain and nervous system to patrol the tissue cells as they do in normal people. The nerve sheath will be gradually damaged in patients who suffer from lack of oxygen.

Eyesight often improves when a Multiple Sclerosis patient has hyperbaric oxygen treatment, because good eyesight depends on a good supply of oxygen in the blood.

All in all we should realise that, whichever method is used, if one Multiple Sclerosis patient benefits, anything should be done to give other Multiple Sclerosis patients also the chance to use this method. Any method should be available to every patient.

Homoeopathy and Phytotherapy

IF EVER I were asked to name a beneficial treatment for Multiple Sclerosis patients, I would immediately answer that there are several aspects in homoeopathy and phytotherapy which are to be recommended.

When Dr Samuel Hahnemann studied homoeopathic principles in comparison to accepted allopathic treatments he reached some surprising conclusions. He started by putting down four basic principles.

First he realised the need to create a mental image of a patient as an individual. He developed a threefold method of treatment, where body, mind and spirit were taken into consideration. These three aspects of treatment are based on the personality and the reactions of the individual.

Next he took the point of view that disease should be regarded as a disharmony. He recommended that the state of the disorder be studied without labelling the symptom according to clinical findings.

He also set out to restore harmony without the use of drugs, which might work short-term, but which often destroy friendly bacteria in the process.

Lastly he intended to investigate the patient's natural defence system to outside influences to which the patient might be subjected. This was in order to build up the immune system, in order to minimise the effects of outside influences detrimental to the patient's general health.

In order to follow these guidelines Hahnemann had to research the Vital Force in all which is alive, and direct this Vital Force according to the principles of homoeopathic medicine.

Looking at the first three lines of thought Hahnemann followed, we understand the age-old idea *Similia Similibus Curentur*, or "Like Cures Like".

Treat the patient as a whole rather than treat the symptoms, was his motto, and always look for the cause of the problem. In this way he arrived at his fourth and concluding principle: to strengthen the immune system.

All homoeopathic practitioners are aware of the fact that if we can rebuild the immune system of the patient, we have laid the foundation on which to continue.

The case of a girl referred to me by a doctor from The Netherlands comes to mind. Although she displayed many of the Multiple Sclerosis symptoms, I was puzzled. After lengthy research I realised from the various tests I had given her, that she had an allergy. The allergy was difficult to pinpoint but it transpired that the birth control pill was the culprit. When I prescribed a homoeopathic remedy to combat this allergy she felt better and the girl's doctor, who later paid a visit to my practice in Scotland, informed me that her walking was continuing to improve.

This explains why so many Multiple Sclerosis patients feel the benefit of a homoeopathic antidote or a nosode remedy if they have ever suffered from measles. In homoeopathy we simply use a rubella potency to remove the miasmas which might still be present from the measles and which influence the immune system of the Multiple

Sclerosis patient.

This can go back for generations, because we have found that even if generations back there had been a case of Syphilis in the family, this could still have its damaging effects. If we use the homoeopathic remedy Syphilinum, we remove the miasma. This is necessary in order to rebuild the immune system of that patient.

Much is written about the use of snake's poison and also how Multiple Sclerosis patients have benefited from the use of Lachesis. Again we can regard this as a delirium tremens, where trembling and confusion is present, and follow the principle "Like cures Like". No small amount of patients who suffered trembling problems have benefited from the use of Lachesis.

When I worked in China for a period of time, I saw how venom was extracted from a snake. Using a hot poker the snake would be forced to spit out its venom. This procedure would be followed in public in the market, where people would be queueing to be served. The venom, diluted with some water or mineral water, would be taken by customers there and then. The relief these people received from a high dosage of Lachesis would quite often be clearly visible.

Each patient should be seen as an individual and having established the characteristics of that patient a remedy should be carefully selected.

Gelsemium, although mostly used for influenza, also gives relief to Multiple Sclerosis patients. One particular female patient was very depressed and although displaying influenza symptoms, was definitely not suffering from influenza. She quickly recovered after taking Gelsemium.

It never fails to surprise me how today's medicine has totally divorced itself from the old way of medicine. Fortunately there is a trend to turn back the clock. The younger medical generation is beginning to show an interest. If we talk about the Vital Force in the human body, having practised in this field so long, we know only too well how easily this Vital Force is disturbed and damaged. We have to go back to nature to realise that one cannot play around with these things without knowledge of the damage which can result.

A wonderful gentle remedy is Ignatia. It will enable the Multiple Sclerosis patient who gets depressed to shake off the damaging clouds of depression.

Zinc preparations have also been of great help to many Multiple Sclerosis patients. Atmospheric influences can do so much harm nowadays. The soil, which once was a rich source of minerals, is now so often treated with chemical fertilisers that it has lost many of its valuable natural minerals. This is all the more reason to emphasise the importance of homoeopathy, with its characteristic absence of side-effects.

In many cases the immune system can be rebuilt by the use of homoeopathic remedies, and miasmas and toxins can be removed. It is also possible to combat certain diseases according to Hahnemann's principle of "Like cures Like". This principle is comprehensible when we think that it is common knowledge that if we are thirsty, we take a little salt in order to quench our thirst, or if we have a cold, we aggravate this condition by sniffing an onion to clear the head.

It is certainly not my intention to write about homoeopathy in detail here. Lots of books have been written on this subject and doubtless more will still be written. I merely stress the point because over the years I have been able to help many Multiple Sclerosis patients by using homoeopathic remedies.

As well as Dr Samuel Hahnemann I would also like to mention Dr Alfred Vogel, whom I would call the man of the phytotherapy. In his time he was practically the only person who managed to convert fresh plants, herbs and roots into diluted form, ready to use. Phytotherapy is sometimes used in combination with homoeopathy, although it may also be prescribed separately.

Hahnemann's principle, to use the Vital Force of anything which is alive, became the foundation of Dr Vogel's work when he started his research with fresh plants, herbs and roots. He managed to manufacture fresh extracts which have been used by millions of people. Many Multiple Sclerosis patients suffer bladder trouble and they certainly do need assistance. Dr Vogel's remedy, Cystoforce, which is a mixture of fresh herbs and plants has brought relief to many and it is one remedy which I often recommend to Multiple Sclerosis patients.

Another remedy of great benefit to Multiple Sclerosis patients is the extract of the Echinacea plant which acts as a natural antibiotic.

The liver is the regulator of our health and as most Multiple Sclerosis patients are plagued with liver problems I often prescribe Boldocynara, an extract of artichokes.

I remember a particular case where Dr Vogel was asked to treat a young man from the Armed Forces who was stricken with Multiple Sclerosis. The three remedies mentioned above were used with good results. Dr Vogel also used the extract of a bull's testicle to rub on the spine of this young soldier, who was able to return to a normal life.

It again proves that one should see each Multiple Sclerosis patient as an individual, with individual needs for treatment. Hence the reason that in this book I have described several methods which may be adapted to suit the individual patient.

I should also mention the remedy Petasan, which almost acts as a cell rejuvenator. This is a remedy obtained from the roots of the Petasitus or pest root, beneficial in combination with some other homoeopathic extracts. A combination of these extracts are marketed as a remedy called MS/55, which contains:

Aurum chlorat.
Beryllium sulfuric.
Cerium chlorat.
Cobalt chlorat.
Cupr. sulfuric.
Ferr. sesquichlor.
Magnes. sulfuric.
Mangan. chlorat.
Platin. chlorat.
Zinc. sulfuric.

I believe that with either homoeopathy or with phytotherapy, whether used separately or in combination with each other, good results may be achieved.

These principles, in accordance with the four principles originally laid down by Dr Hahnemann have already alleviated the suffering of many Multiple Sclerosis patients.

8

Acupuncture

FREQUENTLY I am asked why I think that acupuncture works so well for Multiple Sclerosis patients. In a previous chapter I mentioned that harmony is one of the most important parts in the life of a Multiple Sclerosis patient. What impresses me always when I am in China, is that the three important parts of the great temple in Peking are:

— the supreme temple
— the temple of perfection, and one would say that there is nothing better than perfection. For the Chinese however there is, because the third is
— the temple of harmony.

This is acupuncture in a nutshell. Again in this chapter I will not go into great detail, but I just want to stress a few points, explaining why I am in favour of using acupuncture in the treatment of Multiple Sclerosis patients.

I often ask students to describe in their own words what illness is and receive many different answers. Basically, illness is what the Chinese call "disharmony". We should aim at restoring harmony to that which has been out of harmony in the human body. In the case of Multiple Sclerosis patients there can be quite a few disharmonies.

The Chinese made very sure of three things before I was ever allowed to touch a needle. I had to look, to listen and to feel. They are meticulous in their teaching of what to look for. Look how the hair grows, how the fingernails grow, how the ears stand, for instance. Then one learns to listen to the sounds the patient makes and finally one feels the patient.

What do we feel? Firstly a good acupuncturist has to have a thorough knowledge of pulse diagnosis. It never ceases to surprise me that a very good Chinese acupuncturist will be able to tell how long a person has to live, just by feeling their pulse.

Basically what a good acupuncturist does is to ask himself, after having taken good note of the patient, where the energy in the patient is disturbed. Once we have made sure of our diagnosis we look at the human body as a field of energy. Where disharmony is present we are fortunate that with the help of needles we are often able to restore harmony. We have been taught which points to use, though sometimes a good acupuncturist follows his intuition. He will obtain good results by carefully choosing his points and using his capability as a therapist.

It has only happened once to me and might never happen again, but I never forget a female Multiple Sclerosis patient, in her thirties, who was unable to walk and was bound to her wheelchair. After this patient was placed on the bench I decided where the energy was disturbed and started with the treatment. Afterwards, when she told me that she had some more feeling in her legs and when I asked her to try and stand, she managed to do so. During her next visit I gave her more acupuncture treatment, this time choosing different points, and she managed to walk a little. She again told me afterwards that she felt a little better.

Over such a short period of time one cannot speak of a remission — but there definitely was a sudden change and restoration of energy. I was still sceptical about this sudden improvement, but had to believe it when, on her next visit, I did not see a wheelchair. When her name was called she walked into my consulting room, happy and very much better. She remained very well until she was visited by a neurologist who told her that, although impressed with her improvement, he regarded it as only temporary. Of course this depressed her totally and her husband, very upset, phoned me to tell me that she had slipped back. I had a heart to heart talk with this lady and fortunately after further treatment she improved again.

This again proves that one should have a positive frame of mind no matter whichever treatment one receives or by whomever the treatment is given. Especially when we talk in terms of energy, a positive mind is very important. This lady continued to feel well after her initial slip. I must add that an experience like this might happen only once in a lifetime, but nevertheless it is most encouraging. It also shows that we still know very little about energy.

During question time after lectures, I am often asked what the future of medicine is and generally my answer is that we are only scraping the surface as far as our knowledge of energy is concerned. In our present-day world we need energy-giving foods and we need to learn to direct and transport energy. Anything which can aid a Multiple Sclerosis patient to do that is worth studying. This I often call the future of medicine.

Acupuncture, though often misunderstood, is an ideal method of restoring not only energy but also harmony to the human body. It is God's gift that these energy-restoring points have been discovered. When thousands of years ago the Chinese were fighting each other they became aware of unexpected reactions when arrows hit certain points. This set their philosophers on the trail which resulted in the development of acupuncture. I am grateful that I have been able to benefit from such centuries-old knowledge and study.

In acupuncture we use stomach points, spleen points, kidney points, bladder points and liver points, but it all depends on the symptoms of the Multiple Sclerosis patient concerned which points are relevant to his (or her) condition. With the present electro-acupuncture, very good results have been obtained by treating lung meridians, gall-bladder, stomach and some of the governor points.

The auriculo-acupuncture therapy, which centres on the ear points, is useful in the treatment of muscles, joints, heel, toes, ankle, hip, shoulder and neck movements.

Some Multiple Sclerosis patients suffering from leg spasms I have treated with electrical stimulation of several response points. This treatment, when followed up by auriculo-acupuncture improved their voluntary motor control. This step-by-step programme has achieved some amazing results. It might be that these improvements are due to a change in the extra-cellular fluids, or it might be that the general condition of the patient greatly improved. Although there is still much research to be done, acupuncture used in cases of Multiple Sclerosis is invaluable.

Often I am told by Multiple Sclerosis patients who have been tense and stressed that after acupuncture treatment they feel much better. When the acupuncturist has assessed the imbalance, tensions can be released through use of needles in the chosen positions and gradual improvement for the patient should result.

Every human body has a built-in record of its own life

history and all traumatic events leave a scar which can be systematically identified and sometimes interfered with surgically. Through restoration-acupuncture some life forces can be released and a road to recovery may be found.

My friend and well-known doctor of acupuncture, Walter Thomson, once said in an important lecture that every action causes a reaction. He advised me at the time to use colour therapy in combination with acupuncture treatments. As colour affects us, like cosmic light affects the balance of life, I felt that he had given me good advice. For this reason I occasionally use colour therapy in the treatment of Multiple Sclerosis. This can be carried out at home by the Multiple Sclerosis patient as it is possible to obtain a colour therapy apparatus. The programme to be followed is:

Red Colour

1. The patient lies face down. Start at the base of the spine with magenta light (red and violet). Focus it on the Root Chakram for 15 minutes.
2. Then slowly move it up the spine to the fifth dorsal vertebrae — taking about 5 minutes to reach this part.
3. Focus on the soles of the feet for 15 minutes.
4. Each great sciatic nerve should be treated, allowing the light to play upon the back of the legs in an upward direction.
5. Change to red, treating the knees, shins and feet together for 10 minutes.
6. Switch to indigo. Focus the light for 5 minutes upon the solar plexus.
7. Slowly move the indigo light up to the power centre in the throat. Focus it there for a further 5 minutes.
8. Change to blue and green light for 10 minutes.

If this programme for colour therapy is followed the patient will feel better afterwards. We all know that light affects everything and it can be seen as the activator of life. Sensitivity to light for effectiveness by frequency of colour is an important factor.

As some Multiple Sclerosis patients have used methods such as shiatsu, acupressure or reflexology, I feel that perhaps this colour therapy should be fitted into that particular programme.

In acupuncture terms, it is most important to restore the yin and yang balance when it is disturbed, either anatomically or in other ways. It does not matter if the condition is chronic or acute, the uncomfortable problem is there and needs to be looked at. We are fortunate that this old and proven method is now getting more appreciation in our western world.

9

Enzyme Therapy

ABOUT TWENTY years ago, after giving a lecture in Amsterdam, somebody collided with my car and drove on. I managed to catch up with the other car and, upon approaching the driver, realised that she was very preoccupied. She apologised and told me that she was involved in a difficult stage of a research programme. She gave me to believe that this was a completely new therapy and invited me to come to the factory and see for myself. When I accepted the invitation I had little idea how often I would use this therapy in later years in the treatment of Multiple Sclerosis patients.

I was very interested indeed to learn that the biochemist Mr G H van Leeuwen had developed an enzyme therapy. He set out on the long road of research into all aspects of enzymes and came to the conclusion that many physical complaints could be associated with a shortage of enzymes. He was able to develop an enzyme programme which the human body was able to accept and which could be adapted to the individual problem of a particular patient.

Professor Clausen diagnosed that there were enzyme

deficiencies in some Multiple Sclerosis post-mortems and he also isolated virus infections. There is no guarantee however that this is the case with every Multiple Sclerosis patient. Clausen worked according to the principle that at least three factors should be looked into: Optic atrophy, Intention tremors and Absence of abdominal reflexes together with extensor planter response. Where eye atrophy was present, treatment could be commenced with the enzyme preparation called Oculucidon. This was to be followed with the enzyme Vasolastine and an anti-inflammatory enzyme Rheumajecta. These combinations were to be given together with a follow-up of Coliacron, which is a brain enzyme. In the early stage of the Multiple Sclerosis disease some results are quite remarkable and we have witnessed a rapid return to normal health.

I remember a young Multiple Sclerosis patient who was still mobile, but getting progressively worse. I have looked after her for the past three or four years and, with the help of the Roger MacDougall diet plus these injections, she has been able to maintain her job satisfactorily, has married and lives happily, despite her condition.

Dr Gordon Russell has worked with these enzyme preparations in Great Britain for many years and reports very good results with some of his patients. He quotes the case of a scientist whose eyesight was badly affected and who suffered tremors and had no abdominal reflexes. He has been on the enzyme treatment for many years and has returned to normal health.

Russell also reports on an old lady who has had this treatment for 8 years. She was virtually unable to walk, but now she gets about without a stick and travels regularly to the west coast of Scotland without difficulty.

I will try and explain the enzyme therapy in general and highlight the particular preparations which I have referred to above.

Enzymes are active proteins which bring about all reactions upon which life depends. Enzymatic activities can be arranged in groups according to biological needs.

a. Enzymes which control the metabolism of the neuro-hormones, acetylcholine, adrenaline and histamine. Since the neuro-hormonal system controls the production of enzymes in the whole of the organism, dysfunction can lead to multiple and diverse diseases.

b. Enzymes which control production of the endocrine hormones. Although not directly lethal, these pathological conditions rule out a harmonious development of the individual, either physically or psychically, and they provide the foundation for subsequent constitutional maladies which may lead to an early death.

c. Enzymes of the reticulo-endothelial system, including the synthesis and breakdown of globulins, antibodies, plasma cells and the like. Hypofunction brings about a diminished resistance to infection and hyperfunction is regarded as a likely cause of allergic reactions.

d. The groups of enzymes which produce energy. Inadequate synthesis or disordered activity may lead to dysfunction of all organs and cause many complaints. It may be the cause of the disturbances in all of the above groups. It should also be remembered that the whole metabolism of the cell state is closely connected and, therefore, any functional disorder in one group of enzymes becomes cumulative throughout.

94

There are three alternative consequences of enzymatic dysfunction, depending on the nature of the disturbance:
1. Deficiency or absence of metabolites
2. Excess or accumulation of metabolites
3. Abnormal metabolites
All three are causal factors in a diversity of complaints.

The fundamental principle of enzyme therapy is to treat the primary disease processes of a number of diseases for which, until now, only symptomatic treatment was possible. This makes enzyme therapy a valuable new concept in modern medicine.

The pharmacodynamics of many drugs, including all tranquillisers and anti-histamine drugs, is based on the inhibition of enzymatic functions. It will, therefore, be readily understood that the supply of enzymes, together with their natural activators and inhibitors, into an organism deficient in them, would be the causal therapy for many complaints.

Enzyme therapy enables the organism to combat all illnesses with its own weapons by physiological means. Enzymology is a very complex science and the foregoing brief summary is given as an indication of the many complaints which can result from a deficient or imbalanced enzymatic activity.

VASOLASTINE contains the enzymes which restore the hydrolysis, transport and oxidative breakdown of lipoids and lipo-proteins and thereby starts a 'cleansing process' of the capillary membranes, together with a restoration of brain functions and of the neuro hormonal innervation of the heart and the vascular system. The result is an increased transport of metabolites and oxygen to the organs, and functions which were previously at a low level, are re-activated to normal values. This overall effect is a functional rejuvenation of the organism.

RHEUMATJECTA. The only substances that muscles, nerves and joints have in common are mucopolysaccharides, the principal constituents of connective tissue and of periosteum. Connective tissue is made up of a matrix of chondroitin sulphate sparsely beset with cells. Its function is to lend elastic support to blood vessels and nerves and to detoxicate serum permeating through the connective tissue into the parenchyma. Connective tissue accompanies blood vessels and nerves right down to the smallest branches in the muscles and other organs.

COLIACRON. Disorders in the psychosomatic equilibrium are the source of many pathological developments. Every emotion affects the entire metabolism which undergoes more or less serious changes as a result of these psychic influences. On the other hand, a chronic somatic disease may lead to a psychological change in the patient. The vegetative neuro-hormonal centre in the mid brain is one of the links between mind and body. The medium receives and deals with impulses from all directions, from the centre of the inner life (psyche), from the somatic organism, from the subconscious and from the thinking centres situated in the brain.

It should be borne in mind that the nervous tissue is extremely sensitive to oxygen deficiency. Anoxia leads to irreversible functional inactivations. During nervous activity an adequate supply of oxygen and glucose is imperative for the maintenance of cell metabolism.

Any deficiency in the functioning of these enzyme complexes is removed by the administration of COLIACRON. Disturbances in the functioning of brain and organs and in the development of the functioning of the neuro-vegetative system are favourably affected and removed. An organism which is disturbed in one or more functions, due to physical or mental influences, will manifest the following improvements:

- Restoration of the energy production in the nervous tissue and other organs.
- Restoration of the impulse co-ordination.
- Restoration of the organ innervation, including the hormone producing organs.

Enzyme therapy is conducive to developing the immune system and I would like to elaborate on this ability to rebuild the immune system.

The immune system is a complex matter. The concept of immunity has been extended from the ability to recover or resist disease caused by microbes, to the ability of the body to distinguish self from non-self and to deal with the latter.

There are two types of immunity: the non-specific type and the specific type.

The non-specific resistance is produced by the skin and the mucous membrane, by cells which are capable of ingesting foreign substances caused very often by inflammation, fever or an action of anti-microbial substances. Specific resistance is brought about by the cell-mediated immune system and humoral immune system. The cell-mediated immune system is responsible for its own defence, such as viruses, fungi, protozoans, transplanted tissue and cancer cells. It employs special cells called T-cells. The humoral immune system is responsible for defence against bacteria and viruses. Although it appears that the sole function of the immune system is defence, it also functions as a surveillance system.

The immune system is one of the greatest and most important systems from the day of our birth. To keep our body in good balance it is important to work with any remedies and any foods which will put this immune system in order and so to produce the right energy.

Referring to Clausen's diagnosis on his post-mortem cases that Multiple Sclerosis is often caused by a virus, also explains why the immune system reacts so well to the enzyme therapy. A similar reaction is achieved with Interferon, which is the great new hope and a scientific breakthrough of this century. In some cases of Multiple Sclerosis where other treatments have failed, I have tried Interferon, but because it is difficult to obtain, as well as expensive, it is not within everybody's reach. Certainly in most cases there was a good response and the patients to whom I have given Interferon missed it when the treatment was stopped. In these cases I have been able to trace miasmas of unknown viruses. Initial Interferon treatment certainly builds up our hopes that it will work against viruses and possibly even the slow virus reactions.

If the virus in the system keeps a low profile, the immune system does not come into play and irregularities in the system somehow make it impossible for Interferon to recognise the virus for what it is. If needed the slow viral action is of that kind it will be very difficult to reach.

Some interesting Interferon tests in the United States involved the exposure to the cells of the measle virus. The general feeling is that it remains very important to explore the Interferon impact on individuals in their own medical process. It shows that this potent protein hints at great potential in other areas of medicine, which we are not yet able to estimate.

10

Dental Care

THE TOXICOLOGY CENTRE at the University of Tennessee is known as the best in the USA. In their evaluation of most toxic substances known to man, plutonium is listed as the most deadly, as it is lethal to humans in the least amount known. In an organic consumer report published by Eden Ranch I read that, on the rating scale used at the University of Tennessee, plutonium measures 1900+. Mercury, used in silver dental fillings, on the same scale measures 1600 and nickel measures 600.

Dr Willem Khoe has researched at length how much dental mercury or silver fillings are to blame for further damage to the health of Multiple Sclerosis patients. With the help of several case histories, he informed me that some of his Multiple Sclerosis patients have progressed well after these particular fillings were removed and replaced with composite fillings. This action was followed up with a homoeopathic antidote to mercury.

Since then I have taken considerable effort to look into the effects of silver, mercury and nickel fillings. In my mind there is no doubt that, especially when the patients have an allergy, these fillings can influence their health detrimentally and might even be the cause of the ailment.

An explicit book, *How safe are silver (mercury) fillings?* has been written by Betsy Russell Manning. The book is well researched and well referenced with numerous case histories. She has quoted some really astonishing cases and discussed the matter with dentists and psychiatric physicians.

One typical case concerns a 17-year-old girl who had changed from an outgoing, popular youngster with high school grades, to a recluse, who refused to leave her mother's side. Asked to describe her daughter's behaviour, the mother explained that the girl suddenly reverted to speaking in a childlike manner and tone of voice and displayed an unnatural concern about death. Since the girl had already been seen by about 50 practitioners, including cardiologist, internist, allergist, osteopath, gynaecologist, gyro-practitioner, psychiatrist and psychologist and had been hospitalised for tests, it cannot be argued that her treatment had not been submitted to the best and most expensive. Finally a simple dental problem brought the girl into contact with a dentist who had researched symptoms of mercury toxicity. He thoroughly checked her past medical history and noticed that she had six small amalgam fillings.

Many symptoms have been dealt with in dental and medical papers and journals, singling out mercury, but none had mentioned silver-mercury fillings as a potential or suspected source. Once removal of the silver-mercury fillings was completed, a steady improvement was noticeable.

Until more dentists are aware of the problem, testing will still cause some difficulty as symptoms are not consistent in all patients. A general rule is to start with examination of the white blood count. Other monitored tests include blood chemistry profile, hair analysis for minerals, electro-cardiogram, body temperature, white cell morphological changes, urinary excretion of mercury, whole blood mercury levels, urinary Vit. C, specific gravity and Ph, electrical current (amperage) generated in the oral cavity and other noticeable changes. In some patients changes appear in all areas, but not always in consistent or predictable ways.

After removing dental amalgam fillings and washing mineral salts out of the system, some patients exhibit toxic reactions which have affected the peripheral nervous system, immune system and cardiovascular system. The mercury in the biological system appears to create or mimic many disorders in these three areas, which should be considered.

This report by Manning has given the medical profession something to think about and I am very pleased that in many parts of the world the problem is now receiving attention. Dentists are also taking action by researching into what extent these fillings can have a damaging effect on the general health.

Many years ago when visiting Dr Issell's clinic in Germany, I wondered why he removed all teeth from serious cancer patients. He informed me that he wanted to eliminate in advance any effects of dental infection or of any fillings which might have a harmful effect.

In her book Betsy Russell Manning talks about Dr Voll's system, which I have employed for a number of years, using acupuncture points in the toes and fingers to diagnose dental disease. As a result of this type of testing it is possible to clear up dental problems which are related to the meridians or energetically to organs in the body.

One patient was also mentioned who was freed of his double vision after a wisdom tooth was extracted.

Although this tooth was covered by a gold crown, the real problem was a silver filling underneath. After remedial action this particular patient regained his normal vision.

One of my own patients improved greatly when I used a homoeopathic preparation which was made from a toxic substance and called a nosode for silver amalgam, which was diluted sixfold. After using this nosode there was a reaction and I advised the patient to have her teeth checked thoroughly. One extraction was necessary, after which the expected improvement occurred.

Dr Voll has published a book in Germany in which he lists about 10 or 12 classic homoeopathic remedies to use alongside the nosode for amalgam. Using this method some astonishing results were achieved.

Dr William Boericke, former Professor of Materia Medica of the University of California, San Francisco, has stated that every organ and tissue of the body is more or less affected by mercury. It transforms healthy cells into decrepit, inflamed and necrotic wrecks and decomposes the blood, producing a profound anaemia. The malignant force affects especially the lymphatic system with all its membranes and glands, as well as the internal organs and bones. Even the mind may be affected with loss of memory and weakened willpower. The mouth's salivary secretions are increased, gums become spongy, recede and bleed easily, crowns of teeth decay, teeth loosen, feel tender and elongate.

Dr Willem Khoe, for whom I have great respect, once told me of a Multiple Sclerosis patient who came to see him. This patient had been advised that she had to learn to live with the problems of Multiple Sclerosis. When he examined her teeth, he came to the conclusion that he had to take her off all previous medication and had his dentist remove all old fillings. These were replaced by composite fillings. When the patient was asked for her comment on the treatment, she said that her energy level was up by at least 50% since she began using the device to bring the upper and lower teeth into alignment. She felt that her energy drain had disappeared and that she was progressing all the time.

The fact that people suffer from the Alzheimer disease, which quite often is caused by aluminium poisoning, shows us that these tests cannot be ignored. I have learned recently that some universities in Great Britain are also seriously looking into this problem which, in cases of Multiple Sclerosis and other neurological problems, might be the cause or at least a contributory factor.

The Legislative Committee on Health Care in the United States is conducting a study on the Implants and Therapeutic Devices Disclosure Act. A proposal has been designed to establish the patient's right to know a doctor's responsibility to legislation.

At the 10th Yankee Dental Congress in January 1985 quite a few publications were presented dealing with a review of the present mercury diagnostic services. With some analyses and diagnostic tests these proposals have been proven several times over.

I was asked to give a lecture in Toronto in March 1985, where I was introduced by a pleasant gentleman, who said in his introduction that he felt that we had quite a few things in common. It was not until later that I learned that he was an American dentist who is greatly involved in this particular analysing work. He is part of the Amalgam Toxicity Diagnostic Services in Newton, USA and has found several toxic effects in hydrargyrum mercury quicksilver, displaying itself in symptoms such as allergies, asthma, digestive disorders, skin eruptions, depression, tremors, paralysis, madness, cachexia, etc. Later I listened to a very clear lecture he gave on this subject, from which I quote:

The amalgam toxicity issue, which was dormant for a long time, has been revived again in the past few years. Most of us have been caught in the dilemma between the allegations of toxicity and the assurances of safety. It is a potentially explosive issue, which twice before deeply divided our profession. Mercury, the main ingredient of amalgam, is an element with many unique qualities; among others, it tends to polarise opinions.

In conclusion, some to the obvious facts and verifiable facts:

1. Mercury is a metallic element with unique characteristics. One and a half times as heavy as lead, it is the only metal which is liquid at prevailing temperatures. Mercury evaporates readily, penetrates and dissolves all other metals. It is chemically active and combines eagerly with other elements, forming micro- and bivalent organic or inorganic compounds.
2. No living organism shows physiological need for mercury.
3. Mercury is inimical to life and for this reason it is used in antiseptics, disinfectants, pesticides, insecticides, preservatives, etc.
4. Mercury is toxic and should be handled with caution.
5. Dental amalgam is a mixture of metal alloy with mercury.
6. Amalgam fillings in the human mouth generate unphysiologic electrical currents.
7. Amalgam fillings in the human mouth release mercury vapour.
8. Elemental mercury can be converted to methylmercury by oral and intestinal micro-organisms.
9. Elemental mercury vapour and organic mercury

compounds can penetrate tissue barriers.

10. Mercury accumulates in the body of mammals, including humans.
11. There is no linear correlation between the toxic effects of mercury and mercury concentration in blood, urine, or hair.
12. All the primary scientific research appears to indicate that amalgam fillings can be hazardous to health.
13. Diagnostic criteria used for the detection of macromercurialism are inappropriate for the diagnosis of micromercurialism.
14. Only valid scientific evidence of safety could possibly justify the continuation of amalgam use in dental practice.

I feel fortunate to have been able to meet Dr Victor Penzer, and a good relationship has developed between us. We are both trying to alleviate some of the suffering resulting from these unwanted problems.

11

Exercises, Drinking and Smoking

WHILE PLANNING the contents of this chapter I was consulted by a Multiple Sclerosis patient who has attended our clinic regularly over the past five or six years. With different methods she has been kept going, but she never shows any noticeable improvements. I know for a fact that it is her smoking which keeps her back from improving. She dislikes it intensely when, every time she consults me, I bring up the subject. It is a fact however that Multiple Sclerosis patients who smoke do themselves a lot of damage, not only by the nicotine-poisoning, but also by endangering the supply of oxygen which is so vital, especially to those people.

With so many methods available today to assist smokers to kick the habit, there is no excuse. It is done so easily with the help of acupuncture treatment. The same day I saw that patient, I received a letter from another patient, which read: "I want to thank you for the anti-smoking treatment. Instead of damaging my health, I have now saved enough money to go on a cruise and I am sure that I will not want to spoil the air of the Canary Islands with nicotine fumes, which I now dislike intensely." This particular patient had received acupuncture treatment and was happy, as most patients are according to the many testimonials I receive. I would encourage anyone who smokes, to please seek help if you are not able to stop on your own. It is for the good of your health.

The same goes for the use of alcohol. Under the heading of Dietary Management you have read that certain alcoholic drinks are allowed. Those are the ones which do not contain gluten. From what I have written in the chapter dealing with oxygen, we know that alcohol of any kind affects the liver, which is especially important in Multiple Sclerosis cases. I do know that when Multiple Sclerosis patients get depressed, it is so easy to be tempted, but please understand that with every alcoholic drink taken, you may delay any improvement which might be taking place. Surely it is not too great a sacrifice to give up. There are many other ways to combat depression.

One very much healthier way to achieve relief from depression is through exercise. This will keep you active and at the same time regulate the oxygen supply. Never underestimate the value of any exercises. In my book *By Appointment Only*, dealing with nervous disorders, I have described some very good breathing exercises which not only relax the patient, but stimulate the transportation of oxygen throughout the system.

In this chapter I would like to mention some particularly good exercises for Multiple Sclerosis sufferers, developed by a Dutch colleague of mine who regularly contributes articles to a Dutch magazine specialising in Multiple Sclerosis. These exercises deal with the four main functions, i.e. sitting, standing, lying and moving.

Sitting — Let us first study the effects of the *wrong* posture when slumping in a chair:

107

    a. The head is hanging slightly forwards, which decreases the flow of blood to the brain, thus reducing the oxygen supply. In this position it is more difficult to think clearly or concentrate.

    b. Excessive tension is placed on the back of the neck and relaxes the throat area which is wrong.

    c. The thyroid gland is cramped.

    d. The chest is flattened, which complicates breathing.

    e. The back is rounded, which is unfavourable to the spine and causes extra tension on the back and lack of it on the front.

    f. Resting on the tail-end of the spine could eventually cause haemorrhoids.

    g. Organs in the stomach are cramped and deep breathing becomes impossible.

    h. When crossing the legs, the transport of blood is slowed down in the knee and only one foot is in touch with the ground.

    i. Sitting with crossed arms also hinders breathing.

Now for the *proper* posture:

Sit in such a manner that the seat of the chair takes your total weight. Place both feet on the ground slightly apart. Pay attention to the position of the seatbones, which should be placed firmly on the seat of the chair.

Stretch the upper body and neck and reach with the crown of the head towards the ceiling, inclining the chin slightly towards the chestbone. Relax the arms and shoulders and rest arms on the thighs. Make sure the jaws are slack.

Feel the stomach to check if the breathing reaches down there.

Although it may sound complicated, in time this will become the natural posture. Of the four functions we are dealing with here, sitting should be considered the most important, as a large part of our lives is spent in this position.

To loosen the neck and shoulders we gently and slowly do the following exercise:
1. Lean the head towards the right shoulder as if to touch the shoulder with the ear. Do not raise the shoulder, but keep it relaxed. Repeat twice.
2. Make as if to wipe the ear over the shoulder. Repeat twice.
3. Again incline the head towards the right shoulder. Drop gently forwards, move towards the left shoulder and drop the head back, thus making a circular movement with the head. Repeat twice.
4. Repeat these three exercises to the left.
5. Breathing in, drop the head back, breathing out, drop it forwards.
6. Stretch the vertebrae of the neck while shoulders are still relaxed. Look over right shoulder and turn to face forwards. Repeat twice and do same exercise on the left three times.

After these neck exercises we now concentrate on the shoulders:
1. Pull up the right shoulder as high as possible and then lower. Repeat twice.
2. Bring right shoulder horizontally forwards and then backwards without pulling the shoulder up. Repeat twice.
3. Repeat these exercises towards the left.

Standing — Stand up with the feet slightly apart. Position the feet in direct line with the hips. Relax the knees and place feet firmly on the ground. Achieve the correct position for the pelvis by straightening the spine and stretching the neck.

Make your arms hang down heavily so that the shoulders are relaxed. Jaws also should be relaxed. Oddly, tight jaws may produce tension in the stomach area. Keep the stomach relaxed to facilitate free and easy breathing.

Now we do the "elephant wobble". Shift the weight from the left to the right leg. In this way both legs relax in turn.

Rhythmic movements always have a relaxing effect. With the hips gently make the figure 8 movement sideways.

To strengthen the hips place the feet firmly on the ground and reach upwards with either arm in turn as if picking fruit which is just within reach. Follow this movement through with the hips.

The following little exercise goes to improve our instinctive breathing pattern. Stretch one arm forward and return the arm to the side of the body. Repeat this movement changing arms every now and then. Note that we breathe in when stretching and breathe out when retracting the hand.

Lying — Make sure there is plently of room in order to be comfortable. When lying in a cramped position the transportation of oxygen is hindered. Take up a position on your back with the arms slightly removed from the body, hands and fingers relaxed, feet again slightly apart and in line with the hips. Some prefer to have a small cushion under their knees, the waist or the head. Make yourself comfortable and be aware of all the areas of your body which touch the floor: the heels, calves, thighs, bottom, back, shoulders and finally the head.

Take deep breaths. Move fingers, toes and stretch hands and feet. Make a fist.

Stretch various parts of the body and yawn.

Slowly pull up the right knee so that the sole of the foot

is flat on the ground. Feel the change in the back. Then pull up the left knee. Place right hand under left knee and left hand under the right knee at the back of the thighs (thumbs on the inside and fingers on the outside). Pull your knees up towards the body and gently rock with small movements from left to right. Repeat these movements many times while gradually extending the movement.

At the end of these lying exercises, slowly pull up into a sitting position. Take your time to come out of this relaxed state.

Moving — The same rules apply here as for standing. Models learn to walk properly by balancing a book on their heads. After practice they don't need the book any more: thinking of the book will be enough. Again breathe with awareness.

Another wonderful way to help the condition of Multiple Sclerosis sufferers is with the old method of cold washing. It is recommended to develop the habit of coldwater washing immediately on rising in the morning. Cold water stimulates the blood circulation and the body's activities. Never use warm water when bathing. However, the body and surroundings should be warm when taking a cold bath or shower, thus the body will react to the warmth.

One should acclimatise gradually to this treatment and start with rubbing the body down with cold, wet towels first, starting from the top rubbing downwards. A cold bath or shower should never last longer than 1 minute. Warm water slackens the skin, while cold water spurs it on to activity.

Hydrotherapy is also advantageous in helping defective circulation. A long time back Father Kneipp gave us many good methods of hydrotherapy. I found that a simple way of improving the circulation was a method I learned from an old Indian doctor. This is part of my recommended treatment for Multiple Sclerosis and I refer to it as the "Cold Dip".

This exercise should be done each morning on rising and each night on retiring. Place a basin of cold water with a towel at the side of the bed. On rising in the morning place both feet into the water and count to ten. Then place the feet on to the towel and exercise the toes as if trying to pick up a marble. Do this ten to thirty times. On retiring carry out the same exercise and you will find that your feet are as warm as toast when you get into bed. It is important that this exercise should be kept up for a minimum of 60 days, if you want to feel the benefit. It may look simple, but if carried out properly will have a remedial effect.

One patient came to me after doing this therapy for a little while and was so enthusiastic that he had almost made up his mind that this would help him to solve his problems. Sometimes we see this euphoria with Multiple Sclerosis patients and it could be looked on as a blessing in disguise. Somehow this euphoria helps to carry the patients through the problems of their disease. It also must be a help to their relatives. Patients with euphoria are usually cheerful, bright, and appear happy with their lot in life. They talk a lot, laugh and generally seem happy, despite their physical incapacities and to look at them you wonder what they have to be cheerful about. Perhaps this is God's way of helping to cope.

Despite this exaggerated feeling of well-being in his patients, the practitioner should not underestimate the fact that all treatments should be directed carefully and a proper control of the patient has to be exercised.

Multiple Sclerosis patients could be divided in two groups. One group has this positive and sometimes euphoric feeling, while the other often feels depressed and miserable, making it difficult for the family to cope.

Fortunately the euphoric patients tend to approach things in a positive manner and because of this will benefit from the exercises.

In my opinion one of the finest exercises has been designed by Dr H Moolenburgh from the Netherlands on the basis of the Simonton approach.

First Part — Sit down in an easy chair, with your head resting, your feet flat on the floor. Breathe calmly and hear your breath going in and out. Now take a very deep breath and, when exhaling, say to yourself — Relax! Do this three times.

Now you are going to relax all the muscles of your body. Begin with your eyes and mouth. Squeeze your face tightly together and then suddenly let go. Feel a wave of relaxation travel down your body. Relax consciously your neck, shoulders, arms, hands, stomach, back, upper legs, calves and feet. When you have done this, try to remember a pleasant spot where you would like to be. A lake, a mountainous area, just some holiday spot of which you have fond memories. Imagine you are there and stay with the memory for a couple of minutes.

This is the preparation for the main part of the exercise.

Second Part — Now you are going to see your illness. You are going to *see* with your mind's eye your spinal cord and in this white glistening cord you see some inflamed patches. Sort of gloomy, grey patches that do not look bright, and you are going to *see* with your mind's eye how the bodily defences deal with them. You see blood vessels opening, bringing a flood of healthy blood loaded with vitamins. You see building cells, restoring your fatty layer around the nerve track. If you want to imagine the thing as electric wires being restored, with new insulations being put around them, it is all right. As long as you see with your mind's eye how, with the help of vitamins, minerals and the body's own defence system, the spinal cord is restored to its old function.

Now, when you have finished this mental picture (and you may use your own imagination, as long as you see your illness as *weak* and your bodily defence as *strong*), you are going to see yourself quite strong again. You see yourself walking normally, full of vitality. Pat yourself on the back for having done so well. Breathe deeply three times. Open your eyes.

Do this exercise three times a day: when you wake up, at lunchtime and before you go to sleep. Be in a quiet room. Never skip an exercise. Do not force yourself, just *see* it with your mind's eye. That is enough. What you are really doing is putting a new (and healthy) programme into the computer. It may take you 6 to 12 months before the new programme starts to work out in your body.

Another good way to help the Multiple Sclerosis patient is the Alexander technique, which is a fresh approach to treatment. It cares for the maintenance of health in many conditions classed as neurological disorders, which are given a hopeless prognosis. Even problems like muscular dystrophies and those associated with a repeated trauma, where patients become accident-prone and more off-balance, benefit from the Alexander technique.

It is aimed at the re-alignment of the body framework to the adverse conditions. It is reported that wheelchair cases, who have to exert so much effort to do the simplest of things, have shown great improvement after having practised the Alexander technique. I do feel that if there is an interest in the Alexander technique, the Multiple Sclerosis patient, who usually has the time to do all these exercises, would benefit.

I totally disagree with the often repeated statement that exercises and physiotherapy will do no good for Multiple

Sclerosis sufferers. Many benefit for example from yoga exercises. I have had a running battle with the UK National Health Service about physiotherapy treatment being made available to Multiple Sclerosis sufferers. It is said too often that it is a lost cause and that nothing can be done anymore. The Health Service should provide these methods to Multiple Sclerosis sufferers.

Please take every opportunity to exercise and if your doctor is kind enough I am sure he will do his best to produce physiotherapy treatment. Plenty of good books are written on the subject of yoga and these exercises should also be given consideration.

Finally I would like to mention osteopathy. Although I have practised osteopathy for more than twenty-five years, I do not want to go too deeply into this subject, but one thing always comes to the fore. With every Multiple Sclerosis patient I find that the third and fourth cervical vertebrae need adjusting. A good osteopath should be consulted and from time to time the spine should be manipulated.

Generally I find that a spinal dorsal five adjustment will give relief and also that the dorsal twelve should be seen to, for correct adrenaline supply. From time to time a good massage is beneficial for the circulation. One should however be careful with reflexology, that not too much excitement is aroused, especially when the Multiple Sclerosis patient has muscular spasms.

With all the alternative techniques which are available, there is hope for Multiple Sclerosis sufferers that by practising some of these methods their condition will improve.

12

Conclusion

IN CONCLUSION I would like to list a few general recommendations for Multiple Sclerosis sufferers. The reader
will now have reached the stage of wondering which
course of action to take, considering the many different
methods described.

I have pointed out already that if we have one thousand
Multiple Sclerosis sufferers, we will find that their
symptoms and reactions vary, however slightly. Again I
stress the importance of correct and accurate diagnosis
confirming that Multiple Sclerosis is indeed the ailment
from which the patient is suffering. The treatment may
vary from patient to patient, but there are certain general
recommendations which are common to every Multiple
Sclerosis sufferer.

If a possible cause has been identified, treatment in that
particular direction may begin in order to lay the
foundation for further improvement of the general
condition.

My general recommendation to any Multiple Sclerosis
patient is to follow the four points of the programme

outlined below, which always give a certain degree of success:

1. Gluten-free diet.
2. Supplementary vitamins and use of Oil of Evening Primrose.
3. Hydrotherapy.
4. Acupuncture.

Prior to starting this programme, I generally advise patients to follow an internal cleansing course which makes the body more agreeable to whichever method is used afterwards. In my experience, a good internal cleansing course offers great advantages. Dr Alfred Vogel has developed some excellent herbal remedies, combined as "The Rasayana Cleansing Course" to achieve the cleansing of the liver, kidneys and other important organs.

Fasting is also an ideal way of approaching this cleansing procedure. In the first place we want to cleanse the bowels and through that the blood and the body fluids. It is essential to do this, because our body is affected daily by certain foods, by eating too much or too fast, by pollution of the air, by mental strain and by unexpressed emotions.

When exhausted or over-tired, our body itself produces toxins. We can lose most of this waste matter by exercising in the fresh air, getting enough sleep, deep breathing and not consuming any food after the evening meal (thus fully utilising the naturally available cleaning period). Attention should be paid to life's routine and we should learn to express our emotions better.

The normal excretions of the body take place through the process of sweating, urinary action, bowel movement, breathing, skin scalings, menstruation losses, etc. The four organs responsible for the excretion of waste matter are the bowels, lungs, kidneys and the skin and their actions should be stimulated. Therefore particular attention

117

should be paid to:

1. How we eat. Sit up properly for your meal so that the food receives your full attention. Chew the food properly and mix plenty of saliva with it.
2. Consider your stomach and intestines and try to recognise the first signs of satisfaction.
3. Recognise which emotions take place while eating — if eating creates tension one tends to eat faster, but it might also be possible to release emotions by eating.
4. Be grateful for the food and consider it as a gift from nature. Think of the growing process and of the sun which ripened it.

In this way we benefit from the food we eat and it aids the development of a proper digestive process.

Because of its ability to excrete fluids, the skin is sometimes known as the "third kidney". By using millions of sweat and sebaceous glands, the skin purifies the body fluids of toxins. If one perspires without physical exertion, we receive a warning that there is something wrong. Other signs of high toxicity are:

— an unpleasant body odour despite proper hygiene.
— bad breath.
— bad skin.

For most people the rule can be applied that their own body odour is not unpleasant.

Frequent colds could also be a sign of unfavourable condition of bodyfluids and tissue, which our body does not accept. Therefore we should consider how we can go about cleansing our body fluids.

The toxic matter developed as a result of excessive eating and drinking has a harmful influence. So it is in this area where the cleansing course would be beneficial and there are several ways in which to deal with this. While stringent fasting may only be done under medical supervision, there are less severe ways. For example, the 'mild fast' method designed by Mayr, preceded by a prepatory course.

This preparatory course should be followed for a period of 1 or 2 weeks and the programme is as follows:

1. Every morning on an empty stomach drink ½ litre of water or weak herbal tea, in which a level teaspoon of Epsom Salts has been dissolved. In contrast to laxatives this salt does not irritate the mucous membrane of the stomach or intestines. The digestive system is rinsed and cleansed, thus enabling its own ability to clean itself.
2. Dry-brushing of the skin and morning and evening showers with alternative hot and cold water should be taken.
3. Be aware of what one eats and when, and take a rest of half an hour before lunch.
4. Be sure to take plenty of fluid, which promotes the excretion of toxic matter.
5. Retire at a reasonably early hour.

After this prepatory course, a general improvement should be experienced. Now we go into the cleansing and fasting course, which may be adapted to suit the individual. This course is compiled as follows:

a. Gentle dietary food, with certain forbidden foods and limitations.
b. Remedial exercises.
c. Walking, and if this creates problems, at least spending some time out of doors.
d. Take plenty of rest and take care that mentally one is not taxed.

Of the several methods in use, I would like to pay special

attention to the same fasting method using fruit and vegetable juices.

The principle is to use only fresh and uncooked products. The Epsom Salts should be omitted as they do not combine too well with juices. Juice from fresh and uncooked vegetables and fruit (not mixed) should be squeezed, if and when needed. Proper chewing and salivating is essential in order that the digestive process may start in the mouth.

When the fasting is finished we reach a period of rebuilding. The longer the process is made to last, the better, as the cleansing of the body continues during this process. One could start by adding half a grated apple and some curd or quark, followed by some soft fruit. After some 3 to 6 days a fresh vegetable salad may be added and some grain flakes, and later nuts and seeds.

Try to eat your main meal of the day at lunchtime and drink plenty in between meals.

During the early days one loses mainly fluids, acids and sugars, afterwards also fats mixed with waste matter. These circulating waste products may cause unpleasant side effects, such as headaches, tiredness or dizziness. These are signs that the cleansing course is having effect. To accelerate excretion, plenty of fluid intake, walking and special breathing exercises are recommended. It is equally possible to feel weepy and depressed as it is to feel active, clear-headed and happy. These may all be the effects of fasting, so these emotions should not be depressed.

Although it is an excellent medical therapy, it does not agree with everyone and most definitely if one is not committed to this course of action, there is little point in even starting. To fast successfully one needs to be in the right frame of mind and be mentally balanced.

I should also point out that not every Multiple Sclerosis sufferer reacts favourably to this regime and occasionally an individual will exhibit Multiple Sclerosis symptoms during a fast. As it is not known whether or not these are temporary it is better to stop the fast immediately.

The different attitudes of Multiple Sclerosis patients visiting our clinic is of considerable significance to me. If only they would realise how important is their frame of mind and their ability to look positively at their problem. We then have a foundation on which we can build and accordingly decide on the appropriate treatment.

The only way to approach this illness is to encourage the patient, which in turn produces the best supportive efforts of the practitioner.

In my work I am often reminded of my dear friend Professor MacDougall. The struggle he put up for so many years before finally overcoming his handicap made him a richer person. To look at his outlook on life and his perseverance is to offer a message of encouragement to other Multiple Sclerosis sufferers. Some of his convictions will always stay with me as well as some statements he has made over the years.

— If we fail we degenerate.

— Call it hypoglycaemia, psoriasis or Multiple Sclerosis, these degenerative diseases more or less amount to the same thing. Some unfortunate individual has failed to supply his internal cell-rebuilding mechanism with the necessary ingredients and so suffers the consequences.

— Cell tissue renewal is the physical process of life. The failure to build healthy tissue is just another aspect of life.

— Degeneration is the price we pay for life. Unfortunately nowadays we are attacked not only atmospherically, but also by consuming the wrong

foods and degeneration takes place because of our own ignorance.
— We have to learn the lesson from nature. Realise that we are born part of nature and that we should try to keep nature as clean as possible. The logical conclusion is that we should also attempt to keep our food as natural as possible.

With all the implications of so-called degenerative diseases, it is obvious that we lend ourselves to a variety of problems and that there must be a reason why these diseases have become more apparent in our present day and age. We are responsible for the general well-being of our bodies and we should query and observe where we have gone wrong. Let us join Roger MacDougall in saying that remission is not a miracle. It is due to a logical application of self-evident facts, which have been smothered by a deluge of professional theorising.

I have studied Multiple Sclerosis for more than twenty-five years and there still remain a lot of unanswered questions. If we put all these things together we should realise why Multiple Sclerosis has become so much more apparent in the twentieth century. It is with that realisation that it becomes clear that we have to fight to overcome this crippling illness which afflicts so many people.

It is my sincere wish to assist in any possible way to overcome this problem with the methods already known to us.

Bibliography and Literature

James, Dr P B — *Multiple Sclerosis – Many Scars and Hyperbaric Oxygen Therapy*, Wolfson Institute, Dundee University.

Edelhardt, Mike with **Dr Jean Lindeman** – *Interferon*, Ballantine Books, Ed April 1982

Russell Manning, Betsy – *How Safe are Silver/Mercury Fillings*, P.O. Box 691, Catostoga, Cal. 94515, USA

Graham, Judy – *Multiple Sclerosis – A Self-Help Guide to Its Management*, Thorsons Publishers Ltd 1981.

Vogel, A – *The Nature Doctor* (Eighth Edition 1977), Verlag A. Vogel Teufen/AR/Switzerland.

Horne, Ross – *The Health Revolution* (First Edition 1980), Ross Horne, Avalon Beach, NSW, Australia.

MacDougall, Roger – *My Fight Against Multiple Sclerosis*, Regenics Limited 1975

BY APPOINTMENT ONLY

Dijk, Dr Paul van – *Geneeswijzen*, Uitgeverij Ankh Hermes b.v., Deventer, The Netherlands.

Enzypharm Biochemicals Limited – *A Manual of Enzyme Therapy*, P.O. Box 69, Harrogate, Yorks.

"Uw Richtlijn" – *Publications*, Redaktie: Kapellenberglaan 2, Rozendal (Gld.), The Netherlands.

Index